HIV (AIDS)
Does Not
Mean Death

Volume One

I0113827

Kalu Prince Iroha

HIV (AIDS) Does Not Mean Death, *2nd Edition, Volume One*
"The socio-psychological perspective"

Copyright © 2017 Kalu, Prince Iroha **(MIFSW).**

Email: princeagwu2@yahoo.com

ISBN: 978963255x
ISBN-13: 978-978-96325-5-8

Published by Chiysonovelty International

Further Inquiry: Call + (234) 806 8702 622

Printed in the United States of America

CONTENTS

DEDICATION

This book "HIV (AIDS) DOES NOT MEAN DEATH" is dedicated to God almighty, of whom there is no impossibility.

ACKNOWLEDGEMENT

I am grateful to Pastor Chris Oyakhilome; Reverend Tom & Pastor Joy Amenkhienam; and Pastor Archie & Ngy Aseme, whose love and teachings opened my eyes on my rights, privileges and inheritance in Christ. Thank you my Pastors.

I acknowledge the kind support of my beautiful wife, Hope Prince-Iroha and my lovely children. My late parents; Chief Iroha Kalu Ukoha and Nneoma Nwannediya EziomaIroha are greatly appreciated. My siblings (Rev Omiko & Deborah, Ogba, Joseph, Rose & John, Chukwuma, Nkechi & Sunny; & Chinenyenwa), Rev. Fr. Michael C. Iroh, Rev Evang. NgoziAchike, Elder Nnenna Ojoko, Papa CY, Bros; Ogbusua, Ezema,UkohaIroha, Kalu, Emeka Iroh Elum, Emman, Chidiebere Ume Ph.D, Iya James, Iya Ogadi, Mr/Mrs. Echemazu Chukwueke, Mrs. Grace Iroh Elum, Sunny & Vicky Orji, all Ochoudo, Nde Umezema & Umuokwu family members are appreciated.

My Parents' in-laws, HRH Eze and Ugoeze J.O.R. Ogbuanu; Mr. & Mrs. Alex Njoku, Arc & Mrs. Ejiofor, Mr. Chukwudi John Rogers, Engr . & Mrs. Ikenna Onyemaechi, Pastor & Mrs. Martins Esiaba, Ifeoma, Cherechi, Onyedikachi, the family of Mr. Isaac Rogers; and all my-in-laws are greatly appreciated.

I specially thank Mr. Ignatius Chukwu & family; Barr and Barr Mrs. Ukpai Ukairo Esq. & family; Chan Uche Igwe& family; Chief S. O. Omiko & family; Awa Okoro Nwosu & family; Dr. I. K. Nwagbara of UCTH Calabar & wife Prof (Mrs.) E. N. Nwagbara of Sociology Dept, UNICAL; Dr. Okorie Awa Uchendu, Elder Ndy Okwara, Elder Isaac Abraham, Elder Goddy Okwara, Rev. Miracle Ajah, Rev Kelechi Awah, CP. Ogbusua Aja Rtd., Engr. Ogbonnaya & Ogbonne Ezichi, Rev, Imo Onu, Sam Chiyson Anyaele; Kalada Apiafi, Richard Onuoha, Hon. Chinwe Nwanganga, Endi Ezengwa, Hon. Hagler Okorie, Comrade Isaac O. Isaac, Comrade Sunny Ogele, C.O.T. Uzoaga, Hon. Solomon Akpulonu, Hon. J.O.K. Okiyi, Hon. Kelechi Dede, Gab & Henrienta Oyos, Jeffrey Ebuh, Nkem Joseph Palmer, Kingsley Mbaegbu, Steve Ukiwe, Michael Woryi, UzomaIkoro, Ureh Ireke, Agbai I. Ufere, Harriette & Ndukwe Okorie, Bless Kpai, Charles Osuji, Chidi Imaga, Jason Nwadinobi, Ukadike Ogbuagu, Chibuzor Nwogu, Kelechi Akatobi, Dami Amachree, Anselm Okwara, Sunday Obaga, Joyce Ahuruonye, Egbule Chinedu, Johnson Okorie, Chimaobi Okoro, Ezeifedi Ugonna, Stanley Uzoechi, Kentz Worlu, KC Amadi, Francis Oji, Nnanna Oru Esq, Igwe Olaedo Nwaubani, Opanwa Ikechi, Charles .C. Njoku, Uduma Idika Uduma, Oscar Kalu Nome, Kalu Aso, Chinwendu Ehiemere, Eke Awa Uchendu, Okechukwu Dike Ph.D, Amogu Ukairo, Okoro Awa, Emmanuel Ukweni Esq., Beatrice Nnate, Sunday Olaka, Chinyere Enyinnaya,

Chimaobi Eze Esq., Sunday Iroham, Uche Muoma, Samuel Aso Esq., Uche Emele, Sally Uka Esq., Stanley Mba, Members of Haven D2, Ushers and Members of CC1 Christ Embassy Port Harcourt, Government and good people of Abia State, Staff of Praik-Applied Nigeria, Steering Committee Members and Kids of Abia State Grassroots' Sports Development Initiatives – ABGRASOD, Staff of Wider Perspectives Ltd, Members of Ifemba 3 Age Grade Abia Ohafia, Abia Ohafia and Ohafia indigenes & all my Loved ones who are too numerous to mention.

Thank you for all your care and support; I Love you all.

BOOK REVIEW

Title: **HIV/AIDS DOES NOT MEAN DEATH. THE SOCIO-PSYCHOLOGICAL PERSPECTIVE OF HIV/AIDS: WHY MOST PEOPLE DIE OF HIV/AIDS, (FIRST EDITION).**

Author: Kalu, Prince-Iroha

Reviewer: Okechukwu Kalu Iro

Protocol

PREAMBLE

I was first invited to this gathering as a guest speaker. A few days later the responsibility of a book reviewer was added to me. I wanted to do the two jobs separately, but after going through the book I discovered that what I needed to say as a guest speaker is already contained in the book. There and then I decided to subsume guest speaking in the book review.

THE PREVIEW

I believe the motivation of the Author, Prince Agwu Iroha is the gross abundant lack of interest of Nigerians in knowing their HIV sero-status. As the head of the HIV/AIDS Counseling/ Referral Department of BUNDI International Diagnostics, he was in constant touch with those who stand the risk of HIV infection. Those who are infected with the virus and those who are living with HIV/AIDS. He has first hand knowledge of the result of tests conducted on his client. This more than any other factor, would have prompted him to write "HIV/AIDS does not mean Death. The Socio-Psychological perspective of HIV/AIDS: why most people Die of HIV/AIDS".

The bible says that out of the abundance of the heart the mouth speaks (*Matt. 12:34b*). Prince has seen much and his heart is filled with sorrow for his people. This explains the many words and phrase that he uses for the title of the book. Perhaps a less burdened person would have used fewer words. The entire chapters heading equally portray this heaviness of heart.

PURPOSE OF THE BOOK

The purpose of this book is to expose the reader to the realities of HIV/AIDS in Nigeria.

To achieve the purpose, Prince has four main objectives, namely:

1. To create awareness and educate the reader about HIV/AIDS

2. To convince the reader to know his or her status and, in so doing, to live positively.

3. To reveal to the reader the impact of HIV/AIDS to the individual, the community and the whole nation.

4. To call the reader to action to take up arms against HIV/AIDS and to shun stigma and discrimination against people living with HIV/AIDS.

This review shall look briefly at these objectives.

AWARENESS CREATION AND EDUCATION ABOUT HIV/AIDS.

Prince Kalu devoted the first four chapter of the book to awareness creation and education about HIV/AIDS. From the first chapter he brought his training in psychology and as a counselor to bear by brining the reader to the knowledge of the power of the mind over the body of the sufferer of any ailment, although he feels that HIV/AIDS awareness, education and treatment are given prominence at the expenses of properly examining the socio-psychological nature of the person involved leading to reduced level of success in HIV/AIDS interventions, what he says in the book cannot but add to the body of knowledge of HIV/AIDS which ultimately is education.

Still in the first chapter he goes into poetry to expose to the reader the stark reality of the phenomenon of HIV/AIDS and the absurdity of (casual, unprotected and unsafe) sexual pleasure which leads to life-long pain. At the end of this poem, Prince calls for action to end the pandemic. The action is to get tested, and the second action is to stop stigma and discrimination against people living with AIDS.

In chapter two, Prince Kalu cuts out a large space to

educate his audience about HIV/AIDS. He gives the basic facts about HIV/AIDS and its treatment. HIV means Human Immune Deficiency Virus the epidemiology of HIV/AIDS and its treatment. HIV means Human Immune Deficiency Virus while AIDS means Acquired Immune Deficiency Syndrome. He gives an overview of HIV infection and AIDS, even though all his data at this point were based on the USA and the propounded by the center for Disease Control and Prevention (CDC).

His account of HIV transmission is lucid, emphasizing the main source of infection as sexual intercourse with an infected person, sharing sharp skin instrument with an infected person, receiving blood from an infected person and vertical transmission from an infected mother to her child during pregnancy, at birth, or breast feedings. He allays the fear that HIV could be contracted through kissing, casual contact or insect bites.

There is a detailed account of signs and symptoms; and diagnoses of HIV/AIDS. There is also a section on treatment of HIV/AIDS. Here Prince Kalu demonstrated his ability to do extensive research. He is a social scientist but he delved into the field of pharmacology and toxicology to provide his reader with a list of antiretroviral drugs, their classes, uses, mechanisms of action and side effects.

There is a brief section on opportunistic infection and that afflict the people living with HIV/AIDS.

Prince Kalu has not left his audience without the knowledge of ways and means of preventing HIV infection: abstinence from sex; practicing safe sex-sticking to one faithful uninfected partner, and correct and consistent use of condom; ensuring one receive safe blood; avoiding sharing sharp skin piercing instrument; infected mother submitting themselves to prevention of mother to child transmission of HIV.

The book also treats its reader to myth and the truth of HIV/AIDS and the Global, and national HIV/AIDS incidence and prevalence. The sub-Sahara African bears more than 70% of about 40 million people who live with HIV/AIDS as of December 2004.

He emphasizes the behavioral link of HIV infection. There is also a little exposition on the mode of replication of HIV and how this eventually leads to AIDS.

Window period which complicate the diagnosis of HIV infection in Nigeria is given a section. Prince defines window period as "that period from the time of infection to the time when the usual laboratory test can detect the antibodies to the virus in the HIV infected persons" The importance of other sexually transmitted infection on HIV infection is also highlighted in this chapter.

THE IMPACT OF HIV/AIDS EPIDEMIC.

Prince Kalu sets aside chapter four for the socio-psychological impact of HIV/AIDS. He used the word for death-DEMISE to describe the terminal impact of AIDS on the individual. He recommends pre-and post-tests as an antidote to early death that is currently rampant among people living with AIDS. He posits that a good number of people that have died because of AIDS related diseases did so because of negative attitude to it. He advocates that people should view HIV/AIDS as another chronic life threatening disease whose prognosis can be ameliorated by adequate medical and psychological care.

The impact of HIV/AIDS on the faith communities is also mentioned in chapter four, resources meant for the development of infrastructure and superstructure is taken up by the funding of HIV/AIDS programmes. This is despite the fact that the teachings of the faith communities are clearly against the life style that expose people to HIV infection.

In chapter six, Prince Kalu looks at the demographic impact of HIV/AIDS. He traces the national sentinel survey result of HIV sero-prevalence since 1991 stressing that the worst affected age group is 21 – 29 years. He gives a synopsis of the efforts of the Federal Government of Nigeria at curbing the HIV/AIDS epidemic in Nigeria.

CALL TO ACTION

In chapter six and seven, the book calls the reader to action. The person living with HIV/AIDS is guided how to live positively. The counselor is given some steps to take in HIV/AIDS counseling. The person living with HIV/AIDS who needs Antiretroviral Therapy is given a list of Anti-retroviral drug centers over the Federation.

The author also gives tips on how to care for people living with HIV/AIDS and how not to stigmatize and discriminate against them. He also called for greater involvement of people living with HIV/AIDS in matters of HIV/AIDS in Nigeria.

CONCLUSION

In all, the style of this book is lucid, conversational and brisk. There is an attempt to carry everybody along: the young, the middle aged, the old, the lay person and the professional. The purpose and objective is to address contemporary issues in the global fight against HIV/AIDS. The book shall be of immense benefit to any person who has anything to do with HIV/AIDS including the health professional, the social scientist, the policy maker, NGO person and the individual who wants information. I therefore recommend it to all and sundry.

REV. OKECHUKWU KALU IRO

National AIDS Programme Coordinator

The Presbyterian Church of Nigeria (*2006*)

FOREWORD

In the last two years, I have had cause to work closely with government and non-governmental agencies on the social problem of HIV/AIDS. During these exposures, I learnt that many Nigerians are dying of AIDS without knowing it or because their status had turned to full blow AIDS and as such beyond the reach of available anti-retroviral drugs when they sought help.

I have also come to realize the reason why so many people die of the disease. This is basically due to two main factors namely, ignorance and fear of stigmatization. Most Nigerians still do not know the "ABC" of HIV/AIDS while those who are knowledge about the pandemic are scared to death about going about for HIV test because of its attendant stigma by the society.

Prince Agwu Iroha Kalu has set for himself the difficult task of presenting the phenomenon of HIV/AIDS to the general public as diseases that should be seen like any other diseases like malaria and also directing them where and how to get help anonymously (*especially using a simple test kit in their bedrooms to know their HIV status by themselves!*) In the following pages, you will be exposed to a rich and brilliant discourse on knowledge, care, counseling, etc, about HIV/AIDS. The book is quite a handy phenomenon.

I commend the painstaking effort of this young Nigerian and I do not hesitate to recommend the book to everybody; students, researcher, policy-makers, NGOs who would want to see an end to this dreaded disease in the nearest future.

PROF. EUCHARIA N. NWAGBARA

Department of Sociology, University of Calabar.

ENDORSEMENT

This book HIV/AIDS DOES NOT MEAN DEATH is a radical departure from the generally held notion that once infected, death is inevitable.

The author, Kalu Prince-Agwu Iroha is a professional Social Worker with an enthusiasm to contribute unreservedly in protecting the feelings and health of the society. Everyone; the infected and uninfected has a chance to live, on the condition, which you must take the precautions stated in this book.

This book not only differentiated HIV from AIDS but goes ahead to teach that testing for the virus is the first weapon against AIDS. A home test kit like "Bundi Rapid HIV Self Test Kit" is recommended because the screening result goes directly to the person in quote thereby reducing stigmatization, a risk associated with being tested in a public laboratory.

Knowledge is Power; this book is helpful and a guide to safer sexual relationships. Read this book, help yourself and save the lives of those who depend on you for advice and guidelines. Everyone is at risk.

CHANCELLOR IGWE, UCHE IGWE

I n the following pages you will be exposed to a rich and scintillating cocktail of knowledge on HIV and AIDS.

The beauty of the book is in the brevity with which issues are presented. As you read the last page, you will come to the conclusion that this is a rich poetry in the canvass of AIDS literature. The column of abbreviations is a journey in knowledge.

As a matter of fact, I recommend the book as a good text for the emerging school curricula on HIV and AIDS. What comes out is that the battle against HIV and AIDS can be won. The battle against HIV and AIDS, as you discover is not against the god or demon. It is rather against the weakness of humanity.

In conclusion, I commend Prince for a princely presentation. My hope is that this work is just the beginning of more that will flow from his fertile mind.

UKPAI UKAIRO ESQ.

Principal Consultant,

Nde Udo Chambers.

PROLOGUE

"In too many countries, an official conspiracy of silence about AIDS has denied people information that could've saved their lived. We must empower people to protect themselves through information and supportive social environment that reduce their vulnerability to infections". Kofi A. Annan. Ex - Sec General, United Nations.

A certain lady walked into my office while I was with BUNDI, depressed and looking hopeless. Really, to her it seemed it was over. Mere seeing her, I was able to observe that she was traumatized psychologically. After calming her down, I asked to know the cause of her depression, she opened up to me. Frankly, she tested positive to HIV sero-status test just two weeks before coming to meet me and as she narrated, before her test, she was healthy; after the test, it then seemed to her that she was about dying, hence her haggard look. I understood her problem to be her perception of HIV. After counseling her, I insisted that she should re-test to confirm her perceived status. Though she tested HIV positive after the re-test, I was aware that the state of her mind will not assimilate any negative result thus I told her that she was alright, but brought to her notice that if she is unable to take care of herself, that she will be bound to have AIDS because of the state of her health. She then became anxious to know what to do in other not to have AIDS; she was then referred and placed on Anti-Retroviral drugs. Some weeks later, she came back to me looking healthier and confessing to me that I've saved her life by telling her the truth. She is healthy till date.

The woman in question is HIV positive but would've been better placed on treatment without being told because of her emotional state (that doesn't mean that she won't ever be told as to avoid infecting others and re-infection).

Probably, many may have died because of the psychological trauma associated with being informed that one is HIV positive; why I said this is that, most people prefer to be HIV positive without knowing their status just because of the kind of the impression we have about HIV. HIV is not the same as AIDS. To them, once you have HIV that your days are numbered; which is absolutely not true. These prompted my writing this textbook so as to change these perceptions.

AIDS is real and currently has no cure (though intensive research are on to get one soon), but HIV is manageable. One can live with HIV all through his life span. It's pertinent to state that HIV is not yet AIDS but can progress to AIDS if appropriate measures are not taken.

I personally regret the fact that this second edition of "HIV does not mean death" came out quite belated, the manuscripts have been ready for quite some years ago; but it is an asset to the reader. Thank you.

CHAPTER ONE

INTRODUCTION

"IF YOU FEEL YOU ARE SICK, REALLY YOU ARE SICK".

In a world like ours where human thoughts and feelings affects human actions and reactions, it is necessary to find a way to change most ill-fated feelings before it goes to the extent of affecting the psycho-physiological well being of the person concerned.

If you can reason alongside with me, you will find out that most bio-physical dye-functionality of human beings is due to some socio-psychological imbalance of the people concerned. Typical examples are the cases associated with: stroke, heart attack, cardiac arrest, high blood pressure, low blood pressure; which all results to death or leaves permanent disabilities in the bodies of the people concerned.

These are all related to the ways in which the human thoughts, feelings, attitudes, beliefs, impressions which leads to perception, prejudices, stigmas, stereotypes and other socio-psychological imbalances result to physic-biological dye-functionalities. Sequel to several analyses of scholars as related to the relationship between socio-psychological imbalance and bio-physical mal-functioning in human beings, it was highly observed that the mortality rate as related to HIV/AIDS are mostly related to the socio-psychological depression and imbalances. This implies that if attentions are being focused on HIV/AIDS awareness, education and treatment without looking at the socio-psychological nature of the PLHAs, genuine success would have been compromised.

We can now see that a healthy person is that man who is in total control of his state of mind irrespective of what the situation at hand might be. In the light of the above and in the bid to ameliorate this social problem called "AIDS" pandemic, I've deemed it necessary to write towards changing the conceptions of the members of our society by publishing this text **"HIV (AIDS) DOES NOT MEAN DEATH"**.

"ALL THAT GLITTERS ARE NOT GOLD"

Five minutes of pleasure

A life time in agony

Destiny shattered

Regrets and pains set-in

Could it be fun?

Is fun death?

No, certainly no

Is fun death?

Yes, certainly yes

Five minutes of insanity

That set mind and body at variance

Which brings fulfilling ecstasy

But come with death.

Five minutes of pleasure

Causing pains and regrets

Bringing waste to the body and soul

All through the life time

Putting a stop to great destinies

Tearing families apart

Being like a child

Hiding behind the mother's back

That forces itself into the open door

Five minutes of beautiful ecstasy

Turned into devastating condition

Incapacitating even the strongest man

Thereby causing man regrets his birth.

Five minutes of pleasure

Pleasure, which could've brought laughter

Now turned into an unpleasant condition

Could it be fun?

Fun that has a stamp on the newborn baby

An innocent child indeed

Bringing the past into the future

Exposing the parents mal-functionality

Could it be fun?

As convenient as it seems

Looking good as deemed fit for a lady

Polished nails, alas fun indeed

Fun that leads to death

Five minutes of pleasure

A highway to the grave

Stars have risen for remedy

Likes of Abalaka, Joshua etc.

Did they actually do it?

They tried but couldn't put an end to it

Is anti-retroviral drug the solution?

Not exactly.

Simple ABC methods cum testing

The scourge can be ameliorated

If not, HIV comes knocking

Like thieves who come when guards are down

Becomes AIDS and ends in the grave

Five-minute pleasure

Is it really pleasure?

Without pleasure, still surfaces

Simple mistakes and careless behaviours;

Sharing objects that have infected blood

Who should be blamed?

Nobody, indeed everybody

Deformity cases disability

Africans, it's high time we know our stand

Let's end this pandemic by getting tested

Life goes on

Life is beautiful

Let's stop stigmatizing and rejecting PLWA's

This is time to act.

CHAPTER TWO

HIV/AIDS AT A GLANCE

Human Immunodeficiency Virus (*HIV*) is the virus that causes the Acquired Immune Deficiency Syndrome (AIDS). HIV is a virus that goes a long way to kill the human immune system thereby making the human body porous to aliment and rarely possible to fight certain infections and other mal-functionalities of the body.

AIDS is a condition that makes the body system vulnerable to infections and diseases (Opportunity Infections). I think it will be nice to explain the alphabetical meaning of these acronyms.

HIV STANDS FOR:

• H – HUMAN: This is because the virus only lives in the human beings and not in animals, insects, water, air, etc.

▪ I – IMMUNODEFICIENCY: The virus causes the body soldiers that acts as body defense mechanism not to be effective in protecting the body from diseases.

▪ V – VIRUS: This is a very small germ that we cannot see with our eyes but are very harmful to the body.

AIDS STANDS FOR:

- A – ACQUIRED: This means that one get the disease (condition) from somewhere else and that the body does not make or manufacture the disease.
- I – IMMUNE: This means that one is protected and has body soldiers with the ability to fight illness so that one can stay healthy.
- D – DEFICIENCY: This means that one is lacking something.
- S – SYNDROME: This is a group of infections that happens together. People with AIDS get many of the same type of infection and illness such as cough, diarrhea, skin infection etc.

HIV AND AIDS: AN OVERVIEW.

AIDS (Acquired Immune Deficiency Syndrome) was first reported among homosexuals in the United States in 1981 and has since become a major worldwide epidemic.

AIDS is caused by (Human Immunodeficiency Virus). By killing or damaging cells of the body's immune system, HIV progressively destroys the body's ability to fight infections and certain cancers. People diagnosed with AIDS may get life threatening diseases called opportunistic infections, which are caused by microbes such as virus or bacteria that usually do not make healthy people sick.

As at the year 2012, more than 110,000 cases of AIDS have been reported in the United State since 1981 as many as 1,500,000 Americans may be infected with HIV, one-quarter of who are unaware of their infection.

THE ORIGIN, MYTH OR TRUTH OF HIV/AIDS.

Many people have different views about the origin of HIV/AIDS. For the sake of this text, we are going to see some of the views and then inform our dear readers the widely accepted origin of HIV/AIDS.

Some people are of the view that HIV/AIDS emanated as a result of some biomedical warfare misused. It's also believed by this set of scholars that a similar weapon was used against Ireland earlier before the emergency of HIV/AIDS. But in the Irish case, it was a bio physical weapon in form of milk, which destroyed their fertilities thereby rendering them impotent. From this destructive point of view, it was the reason why the Ireland has a reasonable number of Catholic Priests.

Some years ago, similar weapon came into being but this time around against the Chinese to reduce their population but was detected on time. The severe Acute Respiratory Syndrome (SARS) was detected on time against the Chinese and was harnessed and ameliorated. From this originating point of view, HIV/AIDS was as a result of war weapon emanated by the Americans but was wrongly used thus making it becoming one of the greatest social problems facing the human race. Indeed this view is not widely accepted and is regarded as a mere folktale by the author and several others.

The widely accepted origin of HIV/AIDS could be traced to the year nineteen hundred and eighty one (1981) among some homosexuals in the New York City of the United State of America. *Indeed, the author of this text is one of those that hold this view.*

WHAT IS AIDS?

The term AIDS applies to the most advanced stages of HIV infection. CDC developed official criteria for the definition of AIDS in the United States.

CDC's definition of AIDS includes all HIV infected people who have fewer than 200 CD4+ T cells per cubic millimeter of blood. (Healthy adults usually have CD4+ T cell counts of 1,000 or more). In addition, the definition includes 26 clinical conditions that affect people with advanced HIV disease.

Most of these conditions are opportunistic infections that generally do not affect healthy people. In people with AIDS, these infections are often severe and sometimes fatal because the immune system is so ravaged by HIV that the body cannot fight off certain bacteria, viruses, fungi, parasites, and other microbes. Symptoms of opportunistic infections common in people with AIDS include:

- Coughing and shortness of breath
- Seizures and lack of coordination
- Difficult or painful swallowing

- Mental symptoms such as confusion and forgetfulness
- Severe and persistent diarrhea
- Fever
- Vision loss
- Nausea, abdominal cramps, and fatigue
- Severe headaches
- Coma

Children with AIDS may get the same opportunistic infections as do adults with the disease. In addition, they also have severe forms of the typically common childhood bacterial infections, such as conjunctives (pink eye), ear infections, and tonsillitis. People with AIDS are also practically prone to developing various cancers, especially those caused by viruses such as Kaposi's sarcoma and cervical cancer, or cancer of the immune system known as Lymphomas.

These cancers are usually more aggressive and difficult to treat in people with AIDS. Signs of Kaposi's sarcoma in light skinned people are round brown, reddish, or purple spots that develop in the skin or in the mouth. In dark skinned people, the spots are more pigmented. During the course of HIV infection, most people experience a gradual decline in the number of CD4+ T~cells, although some may have abrupt and dramatic drops in their CD4+ T~cells counts. A person with CD4+ T~cells above 200 may experience some of the early symptoms of HIV disease. Others may have no symptoms even though their CD4+ T~cells counts are below 200.

Many people are so debilitated by the symptoms of AIDS that they cannot hold a steady job or do household chores. Other people with AIDS may experience phase of intense life threatening illness followed by phases in which they function normally. A small number of people first infected with HIV 10 or more years ago have not developed symptoms of AIDS. Scientists are trying to determine what factors may account for their lack of progression to AIDS, such as:

- Whether their immune systems have particular characteristics
- Whether they were infected with a less aggressive strain of the virus
- If their genes may protect them from the effects of HIV scientist hope that understating the body's natural method of controlling infection may lead to ideas for protective HIV vaccines and use of vaccines to prevent the disease from progressing to AIDS.

DIAGNOSIS.

Because early HIV infection often causes no symptoms, your health care provider usually can diagnose it by testing your blood for the presence of antibodies (disease-fighting proteins) to HIV. HIV antibodies generally do not reach noticeable levels in the blood for 1 to 3 months following infections.

It may take the antibodies as long as 6 months to be produced in quantities large enough to show up in recently infected (acute infection), your health care provider can screen you for the presence of HIV genetic material. Directs screening of HIV is extremely critical in order to prevent transmission of HIV from recently infected individuals.

If you have been exposed to the virus, you should get an HIV tests as soon as you are likely to develop antibodies to the virus-within 6 week to 12 months after possible exposure to the virus. By getting tested early, if infected, you can discuss with your health care provider when you should start treatment to help your immune system combat HIV and help the emergency of certain opportunistic infections (see section on treatment below).

Early testing also alerts you to avoid high-risk behaviors that could spread the virus to others. Most health care providers can do HIV testing and will usually offer you counseling at the same time. Of course, you can be tested anonymously at many sites if you are concerned about confidentiality. Health care providers diagnose HIV infection by using two different types of antibody test: ELISA and Western Blot.

If you are highly likely to be infected with HIV but has been tested negative for both tests, your health care provider may request additional tests. You also may be told to repeat antibody testing at a later date, when antibodies to HIV are likely to have developed.

Babies born to mothers infected with HIV may or not be infected with the virus, but all carry their mother's antibodies infected with HIV for several months. If these babies lack symptoms, a doctor cannot make a definitive diagnosis of HIV infection using standard antibody. Health care providers are using new technologies to detect HIV to more accurately determine HIV infection in infants between ages 3 months and 15 months. They are evaluating a number of blood tests to determine which ones are best for diagnosing HIV infection in babies younger than 3 months.

TRANSMISSION.

HIV is spread most commonly by having unprotected sex with an infected partner. The virus can enter the body through the lining of the vagina, vulva, penis, rectum, or mouth during sex.

RISKY BEHAVIOR.

HIV can infect anyone who practices risky behavior such as:

- Sharing needles, syringes and other sharp piercing objects.
- Having sexual contact, including oral, with an infected person without using condom properly.

- Having unprotected sexual contact with someone whose HIV status is unknown

INFECTED BLOOD AND ORGANS/TISUUES TRANSPLANT.

HIV is also spread through transfusion of HIV infected blood during blood transfusion and the transplanting of organs and / or tissues. This was rampant before heat-treating techniques to destroy HIV in blood products were introduced; HIV was highly transmitted through transfusions of contaminated blood or blood components. Today, because of blood screening and heat treatment, the risk of getting HIV from such transfusions is extremely minimal.

CONTAMINATED SHARP OBJECTS.

HIV is frequently spread among injecting drug users by sharing of needles or syringes contaminated with very small quantities of blood from someone infected with the virus. It is rare, but however, a patient can infect HIV to a health care worker or vice-versa by accidental sticks with contaminated needles or other medical instruments.

MOTHER TO CHILD.

Women can transmit HIV to their babies during pregnancy, child delivery, and / or breast-feeding. Approximately one-quarter to one-third of all untreated pregnant women infected with HIV will pass the infection to their babies.

If the mother takes certain drugs during pregnancy, she can significantly reduce the chances that her baby will get infected with HIV. If health care providers treat HIV-infected pregnant women and deliver their babies by cesarean section, the chances of the baby being infected can be reduced to a rate of 1 percent. HIV infection of newborns has been almost eradicated in the United States due to appropriate treatment. But in Nigeria, we still have cases where newborns of (6) six months old are diagnosed with HIV.

Though newborns didn't have their own antibodies, they mostly end up being nurtured with that of the mothers. HIV cases in the newborns are still witnessed in our society today. A study by national Institute of Allergy and Infectious Disease (NIAID) in Uganda found a highly effective and safe drug for preventing transmission of HIV from an infected mother to her newborn.

Independent studies have also confirms this finding. This regimen is more affordable and practical than any other examined to date. Results from the study show that a single oral dose of the antiretroviral drugs nevirapine (NVP) given to an HIV-infected woman in labor and another to her baby within 3 days of birth reduces the transmission rate of HIV by half compared with a similar short course of AZT (Azidothymidine)

SALIVA.

Although researchers have found HIV in the saliva of infected people, there is no evidence that the virus is spread by contact with saliva. Laboratory studies reveal that saliva has natural properties that limit the power of HIV to infect, and the amount of virus in saliva appears to be very low. Research studies of people infected with HIV have found no evidence that the virus is spread to others through saliva by kissing. The lining of the mouth, however, can be infected and it has been reported. Scientists have found no evidence that HIV is spread through sweat, tears, urine, or faces.

CASUAL CONTACT.

Studies of families of HIV-infected people have shown clearly that HIV is not spread through casual contact such as the sharing of food utensils, towels and bedding, swimming pools, telephones, or toilet seats. HIV is not spread by biting insects such as mosquitoes or bedbugs.

SEXUALLY TRANSMITTED INFECTIONS.

If you have a sexually transmitted infection (STI) such as syphilis, genital herpes, Chlamydia infection, gonorrhea, or bacteria veginosis appears, you may be more susceptible to getting HIV infection during sex with infected partners.

EARLY SYMPTOMS OF HIV INFECTION.

If you are like many people, you will not have any symptom when you first become infected with HIV. You may, however flu-like illnesses have within a month or two after exposure to the virus.

This illness may include

- Fever
- Headache
- Tiredness
- Enlarge lymph nodes (glands of the immune system easily felt in the neck and groin), and so on.

These symptoms usually disappear within a week to a month and are often mistaken for those of another viral infection. During this period, people are very infectious, and HIV is present in large quantities in genital fluids. More persistent or severe symptoms may not appear for 10 years or more after HIV first enters the body in adults, or within 2 years in children born with HIV infection. This period of *"asymptotic infection"* varies greatly in each individual. Some people may begin to have symptoms within a few months, while others may be symptom-free for more than 10 years.

Even during the asymptotic period, the virus is actually multiplying, infecting, and killing cells of the immune system. The virus can also hide within infected cells and lay dormant. The most obvious effect of HIV infection is a declined in the number of CD4 positive T (CD4+) cells found in the blood-the immune system's key infection fighters. The virus slowly diseases or destroys these cells without causing symptoms. As the immune system worsens, a variety of complications start to take over. For many people, the first signs of infection are large lymph nodes or "swollen glands" that may be enlarged for more than 3 months. Other symptoms often experienced months to years before the onset of AIDS include

- Lack of energy
- Weight loss
- Frequent fevers and sweats
- Persistent or frequent yeast infections (oral or vaginal)
- Persistent skin rashes or flaky skin
- Pelvic inflammatory diseases in women that does not respond to treatment
- Short-term memory loss

Some people develop frequent and severe herpes infections that cause mouth, genital, or anal sores, or a painful nerve disease called shingles. Children may grow slowly or be sick a lot.

MODE OF TRANSMISSION.

For the purpose of this text, let's view the basic mediums of contracting HIV.

HIV infection can be transmitted through:

1. Having unprotected sexual intercourse with an infected person.

2. Transfusion of infected HIV blood.

3. Sharing of infected sharp unsterilized objects.

4. Mother to child transmission (MTCT).

HIV INFECTION CAN BE PREVENTED BY:

1.   Abstinence from sex

2.   Practicing safe sex: stick to one faithful uninfected partner, don't practice unprotected sex.

3.   Ensuring that you receive only screened HIV negative blood.

4.   Avoiding the use of unsterilized skin piercing instruments/sharing piercing objects.

5.   Infected mothers seeking advice before pregnancy, drug therapy, breast feeding and delivery options may have to be considered.

6.   If you can't adhere to abstinence, then ensure that you use condom of approved quality properly and consistently.

SYMPTOMS

The best way to know whether one has HIV or not is through HIV antibody screening. This is because HIV has no signs or symptoms rather AIDS does. The concept of Signs and Symptoms precipitates as a result of the progression of HIV to AIDS.

These are some of the signs and symptoms associated to the progression of the virus:

▪   Weight loss.
▪   Severe Cough for more than one month.

- Diarrhea lasting for more than one month.
- Acute and severe fatigue.
- Ulcers/ infections
- Night Sweat at all times
- Glands Heats

It is worthwhile to explain here that many of these signs and symptoms are also of other illnesses so the only way to determine it as HIV is through blood test.

CHAPTER THREE

HIV ANALYSIS (ADVANCED ANALYSIS)

BIO-PHYSIOLOGICAL ANALYSIS

As already explained, HIV stands for "Human Immunodeficiency Virus" and it is the virus that progresses to Acquired Immune Deficiency Syndrome (AIDS). HIV is a Virus that people pass to others through blood to-blood or sexual contact. Blood, semen vaginal fluid, and other body fluids that contain blood are all known ways to spread HIV. Pregnant woman can also pass HIV to their babies during pregnancy, during delivery, as well as through breast-feeding.

The most common means of transmission of HIV is sexual intercourse which includes Anal, Oral and Vaginal intercourse with an infected partner. Activities such as unprotected homosexual intercourse or sharing contaminated needles for drug use can also put a risk of contracting HIV. Another less common ways is through blood transfusion and organ or tissue transplants.

You cannot contact HIV through casual contact such a sharing a glass with someone who is HIV positive or using the same toilet with the person. Contact with saliva, sweat, or tears cannot transmit, HIV cannot be transmitted through swimming pool and hot tubs. Since HIV can only live on human cells; pets and insects cannot transmit the virus from an HIV-positive to a non-HIV positive person.

It is very important to note that if you have HIV, it does not necessarily mean that you are sick. It sometimes take years for HIV to progress to AIDS. During this time, people who have HIV can live normal and productive lives.

LIFE CYCLE OF HIV INFECTION

HIV begins with infection of susceptible host cell by binding to the CD4+ receptor on the host cell. CD4+ is present on the surface of many lymphocytes, which is a critical part of the body's immune system. Recent evidence indicates that a co-receptor is needed for HIV to enter the cell. This recognition of HIV co-receptor and progress in understanding how HIV fuses with the cell has opened up new possibilities for ARV. A number of new agents are being designed to prevent infection by blocking fusion of HIV with its host cell following fusion of the virus with the host cell, HIV enters the cell. The genetic material of the virus (RNA) is released and undergoes reverse transcription into DNA.

An enzyme in HIV called Reverse transcriptase is necessary to catalyze this conversion of Viral RNA into DNA. Inhibitors of reverse transcriptase, such as ATZ, were the first anti-HIV medications, and are still a critical part of treating patients who have HIV, reverse transcriptase inhibitors are divided into two classes: nucleoside analogues and non-nucleoside reverse transcriptase inhibitors, this is based on their structure and how they transcriptase.

Once the genetic materials of HIV have been changed into DNA, this Viral DNA enters the host cell nucleus where it can be integrated into the genetic material of the cell. The enzyme **"integrase"** catalyzes this process and inhibitor of integrase is a new way to block HIV replication.

Once the DNA is integrated into the genetic material of the host it possibly may persist in latent state for many years. Those with ability of HIV to persist in certain latently infected cells are the major barrier to eradication or cure of HIV. Activation of the host cells result in the transcription of the DNA into messenger RNA (m RNA) when translated into viral proteins. The Viral RNA and viral protein assemble at the cell membrane into a new virus. Amongst the viral proteins is HIV protease, which requires the process of other HIV proteins to coerce into their functional forms protease inhibitors, one of the most potent types of anti-viral medication, act surface, the virus then buds forth the cell and is released to infect other cells.

THE CONNNECTION BETWEEN HIV/AIDS

HIV is the "Human Immunodeficiency Virus". It is the virus that eventually leads to "Acquired Immune Deficiency Syndrome" (AIDS). Most PLWAs eventually develop AIDS because the virus makes it difficult for the human body to fight off diseases. AIDS is not one sickness, rather a name of a condition that encompasses many illnesses. You can't tell when a person has HIV. A person who is positive can look and feel as healthy as a person who does not have the virus. But when a person who is HIV positive develops AIDS, the person does not only look sick. He or she feels sick; disease takes over the body because HIV has broken down the body's defense mechanism (immune system). These diseases are called opportunistic infection (Ols). They are called Opportunistic Infection because when the body's resistance is weak, infections of all types use the "opportunity" to invade and take over the body. Persons don't actually die of AIDS. Death usually comes after a series of illnesses and when the body finally succumbs to one or more of the diseases, which take over in the AIDS stage.

People living with HIV and AIDS live their lives as usual, but taking extra care of their health; persons with AIDS may be sick too often. To be able to carry on normally, they need care and medical treatment.

THE WINDOW PERIOD

The window period is that period from the time of infection to the time when the usual laboratory test can detect the antibodies of the Virus in the HIV infected person. The window period can last between two weeks to six months. Different people take different length of time to produce and release the antibodies, sometime called "clue" to the Virus.

During the window period, the commonly used tests cannot detect the antibodies to the virus.

Therefore, if someone is tested during that period, the tests result will be negative even though he/she is infected. Some laboratories described the finding as "non-reactive". During the window period an infected person may still infect others if he/she indulges in risky behaviours with uninfected partner(s).

During the window period, the Virus gears capturing the CD4+ cells. The CD4+ itself can only be captured through a co-receptor cell known as the CCR5 Cell.

Researchers have proved that not all human beings have CCR5 Cells. Because of these, it will be difficult for the virus to capture a body system that has no CCR5 Cell. Most times, the virus dies in the body system if its effort to capture the CCR5 cell is fruitless.

We have known cases where the wife is HIV positive while her husband is HIV Negative. Who knows, maybe the husband might have been the one that infected the wife with HIV at the window period but because he doesn't have CCR5 cell in his system, the HIV choked itself to death; thus he ended up not having the virus. In the contrary, the wife has the CCR5 cell, which is the gateway to the CD4+ cell, so she ends up having the virus.

The CD4+ cell and CCR5 cell are issue to be discussed at the next edition of this research work.

WHY ARE SEXUALLY TRANSMITTED INFECTIONS (STIs) IMPORTANTS IN HIV PREVENTION?

Sexually Transmitted Infections (STIs) are transmitted in the same way as HIV. STIs put additional stress on the body's resistance. They create small sores. (Sometimes even invisible) sores on the genitals. These opening may allow HIV to be transmitted easily to the person that has the STIs.

WHO IS AT RISK?

Given the mode of transmission, everyone is at risk. However there are particular behaviours and practices that increase the risk of HIV infection. Such behaviours include:

1.   Having multiple sexually partners whose HIV statuses are unknown.

2.   Engaging in unprotected sex.

3.   Sharing skin-piercing or Drug injection equipment.

4.   Receiving unscreened blood.

IS IT NECESSARY FOR COUPLES TO USE CONDOMS IF THEY ARE BOTH INFECTED WITH HIV?

Yes, if one or both married couple is/are infected, they

should use condom every time they have sex because:

1.   They may be infected with different types of the virus and cross infection may result if condom is not used.

2.   More viruses can be transmitted which may accelerated the onset of AIDS.

HIV ANALYSIS (ADVANCED ANALYSIS) 2

SOCIO-PHYCHOLOGICAL ANALYSIS

"THE GREATEST WAR IS THE WAR AGAINST ONESELF. IF YOU CAN CONTROL YOUR EMOTION, YOU ARE A WINNER".

Unlike the bio-physiological analysis of HIV, the socio-psychological analysis of HIV/AIDS has to do with how and what causes the demise of most PLHAs. Most people condemned themselves once they observed that they are HIV positive. Most people are still with the perception that HIV has no cure which simply means that the carrier's days in the world are numbered. Most people still see HIV from the negative perspective thus prompts the early demise of people that have HIV. Most people still don't believe that HIV is manageable. Indeed, all the above mentioned facts hasten the early demise of the people living with HIV/AIDS.

As said earlier in the preamble, the young lady that I had the encounter with was about dying. Remember, she wasn't sick when she went for the HIV antibody sero-status test. She was just about settling down with her intended spouse when she discovered that she had HIV. The health care provider compounded her case by not counseling her well (he / she could have educate her well on what HIV is all about) before and after the HIV screening. The doctor would've also assessed her emotional state before releasing the result to her. Indeed, most people's emotional states are not matured to assimilate negative HIV test result. These also hasten the progression from HIV to AIDS and enhance the mortality rate as related to HIV.

Before I got established on the HIV counseling profession, I once had a client who slapped me because I told him the bitter truth which was that he was positive. By then, I still had in mind that people's mode of perception was all the same as mine thus prompted my telling him the frank truth in the processing of his HIC Counseling and Testing (HCT).

It will be pertinent to state categorically that it's never a crime to have HIV. Most people who are wayward and promiscuous are not even infected with the virus. Some people who have just had sex for few times are infected and even virgins / faithful partners are infected too. Does it now mean that the latter are more wayward than the former? No. the issue of HIV infection depends on the level of your knowledge about HIV/AIDS prevention and management. HIV/AIDS is in respectable home, Mosques,

Churches, Schools, Banks, and other respected organizations. This now makes HIV/AIDS to be one of the greatest problems that face the entire human race (even though there are still denials on death caused by HIV/AIDS in other to protect the family / organizational names).

It's high time we brought to our respective minds the fact that HIV is not what most people consider it to be *(Please I am not saying that HIV/AIDS is not real).* Rather what I am trying to say is that our mode of perception about HIV which was because of the impression given to us by the World Health Organization is not so. Those infected with HIV stand the same risk with those having High BP, Stroke, Diabetics, Cancers, Asthma etc.

They all have to take care of themselves regularly in order to prolong their respective lives. Then, why is it that those with HIV do not believe that they stand the chance of taking care of themselves and by so doing, prevent or delay the progression to AIDS?

After series of research, it came to my knowledge that people are afraid of going for HIV sero-status test. Why is it so? It is because of the level of our societal understanding of HIV/AIDS. Our society have rated HIV to an extent that whoever that observed that he/she is infected is bound to condemn himself. Really, it's not supposed to be so. HIV is a viral infection just like most other infections. But the peculiar thing with HIV (aside its physiological make-up) is that it is widely believed to have no cure. But you will agree with me that HIV is not the only condition that has no cure. Why then is it highly termed to be the deadliest condition when we still have other conditions that have no physiologically well-diagnosed therapies? It frightens me seeing people with this misconception.

A good number of people that have died as a result of HIV/AIDS died not because of the diseases itself but their death were due to the trauma associated with being HIV positive (which is as a result of the societal stereotype, stigma and label on the concept of HIV/AIDS). Once a person observed that he is infected with HIV, his state of mind is bound to change thereby making his body more porous than what the virus would've made it to be.

One rich young man came to me 6 years ago and was narrating his ordeals to me. It was a sad one indeed. He got a new lady in his life and decided to marry her. Already, he knew his HIV status. He told the lady to go for HIV test. The lady tested positive to HIV antibody sero-status test. She went for a confirmatory test and was positive too, then the man now considered himself to have the virus but still at the window state because he had previously indulged in unprotected sexual intercourse with the lady in question. He then decided to stop the establishment of a business firm which he was handling. What I am saying is that, the young man condemned himself already without confirming whether he is positive or not, but let's assume that he eventually become positive. Should that now be a reason for him to destroy his life even before the virus start destroying him? What I'm saying here is that, most people are just killing themselves just because they tested positive. It shouldn't be so. The essence of this text is to re-orientate the members of our society with respect to their perception of HIV/AIDS and related issues. It is really wise to go for HIV sero-status test so as to know your status. This will, to a large extent, help one to keep himself going, whether he is positive or not. If you know your status you will caution yourself more as regards to the kind of risky behaviour you will be indulging in so as to live a healthy life. HIV/AIDS is real but its epidemic level is being aggravated by our societal perception towards it.

RELIGION (FAITH BASED) ANALYSIS

AIDS is affecting the religious community in many ways. First, many of the PLWAS are religious people, members of churches and mosques. Anything affecting the people of the region affects the region itself. Secondary, resources Building Projects that religious organizations are involved with and activities that need to be developed are usually postponed or cancelled because the funds are being used to care for PLWAS. People who use to devote time in religious activities are now involved in caring for PLWA. Third, AIDS even touches the lives of religious leaders. Nearly every seminary in Jos has lost someone to AIDS in recent Six years ago, Associate Professor Danny McCain of the department of religious studies, University of Jos conducted an AIDS training workshop for teachers of religious studies in Gombe State. Within four months, two of the eighty teachers had become sick of AIDS. Even religious teachers are not exempted from AIDS.

I believe that religious communities have a serious role to play in HIV/AIDS amelioration. The faith based communities have significant contributions to male in many areas of the AIDS-battle.

Both Christian and Islamic Religious bodies have their respective faith-based organizations. For instance; the Presbyterian AIDS at Aba (preby-AIDS), the Catholic Church AIDS group at the Catholic Church Headquarters Durumi Abuja and so on.

The following of the 9 AIDS groups) with based group are not really very easy ventures. These monies as well would've been used for development of the Churches and so on. But they are now diverted towards curbing the HIV/AIDS pandemic.

Really, most International Donor group such as United State Agency for International Development (USAID), United Nation Agency for International Development (UNAIDS), DFID, Food foundation, pathfinder International etc. are helpful to these Religious AIDS groups.

AFRICA AND THE FAITH BASED

Recognizing and worshiping a Divine Being is a universal experience of all Cultures. Though rationalism has undermined some of the religious Commitment in the Western World and Atheism inspired by communism has negatively impacted religions in other part of the world. John Mbiti, a Kenyan expert on Africa Traditional Religion, once said, "Africans are notoriously religious". When Islam came to Africa, it did not meet a religion vacuum. Religion is practiced publicly in Africa. Muslims interrupt their daily activities five times a day to pray and they do so publicly if necessary. Most public gathering are opened and closed with prayer. African languages have been deeply impacted by religion and are filled with blessings, prayers and thanksgivings to God. A very large percentage of names in Africa are connected with God.

Because religion deals with one's perception of the Creator and Owner of the universe, most people take their religion seriously. The foundation of morality is religion. To say it this way, a culture gets its understanding of right and wrong primarily from its religion.

Even the person who claims to practice no religion recognizes that religious beliefs and practices provide stability, order and justice in society. One of the areas of morality that adherents of Christianity and Islam feel especially strongly about is the issue of sexual morality. One of the Ten Commandments in the Holy Bible says "you should not commit adultery" (Exodus 20:14). The Holy Qur'an says "nor come nigh to adultery; for it is an indecent (deed) and evil way" (Al-Israi, Q. 17:32). In fact both the sacred books are filled with examples and instructions about improper use of sexuality.

Immoral sexual behavior is the biggest means of transmitting HIV. It is estimated that over 80% of HIV infections in Africa have come through heterogeneous sexual contact. Therefore, teaching and encouraging people to practice the religious principles related to sex will greatly assist in preventing the spread of HIV transmission.

It will be unfair to discuss these, without mentioning the roles of the religious bodies because they have lots of roles to play towards the prevention and management of HIV.

CHAPTER FOUR

THE DIFFERENT STAGES OF HIV INFECTION

H IV infects cells in the immune system and the central nervous system. The main type of cell that HIV infects is the T helper lymphocyte. These cells play a crucial role in the immune system, by coordinating the actions of other immune system cells. A large reduction in the number of T helper cells seriously weakens the immune system.

HIV infects the T helper cell because it has the protein CD4 on its surface, which HIV uses to attach itself to the cell before gaining entry. This is why the T helper cell is sometimes referred to as a CD4+ lymphocyte. Once it has found its way into a cell, HIV produces new copies of itself, which can then go on to infect other cells.

Over time, HIV infection leads to a severe reduction in the number of T helper cells available to help fight disease. The process usually takes several years.

HIV infection can generally be broken down into four distinct stages: primary infection, clinically asymptomatic stage, symptomatic HIV infection, and progression from HIV to AIDS.

STAGE 1: Primary HIV Infection

This stage of infection lasts for a few weeks and is often accompanied by a short flu-like illness. In up to about 20% of people the symptoms are serious enough to consult a doctor, but the diagnosis of HIV infection is frequently missed.

During this stage there is a large amount of HIV in the peripheral blood and the immune system begins to respond to the virus by producing HIV antibodies and cytotoxic lymphocytes. This process is known as seroconversion. If an HIV antibody test is done before seroconversion is complete then it may not be positive.

STAGE 2: Clinically Asymptomatic Stage

This stage lasts for an average of ten years and, as its name suggests, is free from major symptoms, although there may be swollen glands. The level of HIV in the peripheral blood drops to very low levels but people remain infectious and HIV antibodies are detectable in the blood, so antibody tests will show a positive result.

Research has shown that HIV is not dormant during this stage, but is very active in the lymph nodes. A test is available to measure the small amount of HIV that escapes the lymph nodes. This test which measures HIV RNA (HIV genetic material) is referred to as the viral load test, and it has an important role in the treatment of HIV infection.

STAGE 3: *Symptomatic HIV Infection*

Over time the immune system becomes severely damaged by HIV. This is thought to happen for three main reasons:

- The lymph nodes and tissues become damaged or 'burnt out' because of the years of activity;
- HIV mutates and becomes more pathogenic, in other words stronger and more varied, leading to more T helper cell destruction;
- The body fails to keep up with replacing the T helper cells that are lost.

As the immune system fails, so symptoms develop. Initially many of the symptoms are mild, but as the immune system deteriorates the symptoms worsen.

Where do opportunistic infections and cancers occur?

Symptomatic HIV infection is mainly caused by the emergence of opportunistic infections and cancers that the immune system would normally prevent. These can occur in almost all the body systems, but common examples are featured in the table below.

As the table below indicates, symptomatic HIV infection is often characterised by multi-system disease. Treatment for the specific infection or cancer is often carried out, but the underlying cause is the action of HIV as it erodes the immune system. Unless HIV itself can be slowed down the symptoms of immune suppression will continue to worsen.

System	Examples of Infection/ Cancer
Respiratory system	• Pneumocystis jirovecii Pneumonia (PCP) • Tuberculosis (TB) • Kaposi's Sarcoma (KS)
Gastro-intestinal system	• Cryptosporidiosis • Candida • Cytomegolavirus (CMV) • Isosporiasis • Kaposi's Sarcoma
Central/peripheral Nervous system	• HIV • Cytomegolavirus • Toxoplasmosis • Cryptococcosis • Non Hodgkin's lymphoma • Varicella Zoster • Herpes simplex Skin: Herpes simplex • Kaposi's sarcoma • Varicella Zoster

STAGE 4: Progression from HIV to AIDS

As the immune system becomes more and more damaged the illnesses that occur become more and more severe leading eventually to an AIDS diagnosis.

At present in the UK an AIDS diagnosis is confirmed if a person with HIV develops one or more of a specific number of severe opportunistic infections or cancers. In the US, someone may also be diagnosed with AIDS if they have a very low count of T helper cells in their blood. It is possible for someone to be very ill with HIV but not have an AIDS diagnosis.

WHO clinical staging of HIV disease in adults and adolescents (2013 revision)

In resource-poor communities, medical facilities are sometimes poorly equipped, and it is not possible to use CD4 and viral load test results to determine the right time to begin antiretroviral treatment. The World Health Organisation (WHO) has therefore developed a staging system for HIV disease based on clinical symptoms, which may be used to guide medical decision making.

Clinical Stage I:

- Asymptomatic
- Persistent generalized lymphadenopathy

Clinical Stage II:

- Moderate unexplained weight loss (under 10% of presumed or measured body weight)
- Recurrent respiratory tract infections.
- Herpes zoster
- Angular chelitis

- Recurrent oral ulceration
- Papular pruritic eruptions
- Seborrhoeic dermatitis
- Fungal nail infections

Clinical Stage III:

- Unexplained severe weight loss (over 10% of presumed or measured body weight).
- Unexplained chronic diarrhea for longer than one month
- Unexplained persistent fever (intermittent or constant for longer than one month)
- Persistent oral candidiasis
- Oral hairy leukoplamia
- Pulmonary tuberculosis
- Severe bacterial infections (e.g. pneumonia, empyema, pyomyositis, bone or joint infection, meningitis, bacteraemia)
- Acute necrotizing ulcerative stomatitis, gingivitis or periodontitis
- Unexplained* anaemia (below 8 g/dl), neutropenia (below 0.5 billion/l) and/or chronic thrombocytopenia (below 50 billion/l)

Clinical Stage IV:

- HIV wasting syndrome
- Pneumocystis pneumonia
- Recurrent severe bacterial pneumonia

- Chronic herpes simplex infection (orolabial, genital or anorectal of more than one month's duration or visceral at any site)
- Oesophageal candidiasis (or candidiasis of trachea, bronchi or lungs)
- Extrapulmonary tuberculosis
- Kaposi sarcoma
- Cytomegalovirus infection (retinitis or infection of other organs)
- Central nervous system toxoplasmosis
- HIV encephalopathy
- Extrapulmonary cryptococcosis including meningitis
- Disseminated non-tuberculous mycobacteria infection
- Progressive multifocal leukoencephalopathy
- Chronic cryptosporidiosis
- Chronic isosporiasis
- Disseminated mycosis (extrapulmonary histoplasmosis, coccidiomycosis)
- Recurrent septicaemia (including non-typhoidal Salmonella)
- Lymphoma (cerebral or B cell non-Hodgkin)
- Invasive cervical carcinoma
- Atypical disseminated leishmaniasis
- Symptomatic HIV-associated nephropathy or HIV-associated cardiomyopathy

CHAPTER FIVE

HIV AND AIDS IN NIGERIA

UNAIDS estimates that in Nigeria, around 3.1 percent of adults between ages 15-49 are living with HIV and AIDS. Although the HIV prevalence is much lower in Nigeria than in other African countries such as South Africa and Zambia, the size of Nigeria's population (around 138 million) meant that by the end of 2007, there were an estimated 2,600,000 people infected with HIV.

Approximately 170,000 people died from AIDS in 2007 alone[2]. With AIDS claiming so many people's lives, Nigeria's life expectancy has declined. In 1991 the average life expectancy was 53.8 years for women and 52.6 years for men. In 2007 these figures had fallen to 46 for women and 47 for men.

Despite being the largest oil producer in Africa and the 12th largest in the world[4], Nigeria is ranked 158 out of 177 on the United Nations Development Programme (UNDP) Human Poverty Index. This poor economic position has meant that Nigeria is faced with huge challenges in fighting its HIV/AIDS epidemic.

The history of HIV and AIDS in Nigeria

The first two HIV cases in Nigeria were identified in 1985 and were reported at an international AIDS conference in 1986. In 1987 the Nigerian health sector established the National AIDS Advisory Committee, which was shortly followed by the establishment of the National Expert Advisory Committee on AIDS (NEACA).

At first the Nigerian government was slow to respond to the increasing rates of HIV transmission and it was only in 1991 that the Federal Ministry of Health made their first attempt to assess the Nigerian HIV/AIDS situation. The results showed that around 1.8 percent of the population of Nigeria was infected with HIV. Subsequent surveillance reports revealed that during the 1990s the HIV prevalence rose from 3.8% in 1993 to 4.5% in 1998.

When Olusegun Obasanjo became the president of Nigeria in 1999, HIV/AIDS prevention, treatment and care became one of the government's primary concerns. The President's Committee on AIDS and the National Action Committee on AIDS (NACA) were created, and in 2001, the government set up a three-year HIV/AIDS Emergency Action Plan (HEAP). In the same year, Obasanjo hosted the Organisation of African Unity's first African Summit on HIV/AIDS, Tuberculosis, and Other Related Infectious Diseases.

Despite these positive intentions for tackling the epidemic, in 2006 it was estimated that just 10 percent of HIV-infected women and men were receiving antiretroviral therapy and only 7 percent of pregnant women were receiving treatment to reduce the risk of mother-to-child transmission of HIV.

How is HIV transmitted in Nigeria?

Some 80% of HIV infections in Nigeria are transmitted through heterosexual sex. Factors contributing to this include a lack of information about sexual health and HIV, low levels of condom use and high levels of sexually transmitted infections (STIs) such as chlamvdia and gonorrhoea, which make it easier for the virus to be transmitted.

It has been reported that blood transfusions account for up to 10 percent of new HIV infections in Nigeria. There is a high demand for blood because of blood loss from surgery and childbirth, road-traffic accidents and anaemia and malaria. Not all Nigerian hospitals have the technology to effectively screen blood and therefore contaminated blood is often used. The Nigerian Federal Ministry of Health have responded by backing legislation that requires hospitals to only use blood from the National Blood Transfusion Service, which has far more advanced blood-screening technology.

The other main transmission route is mother-to-child transmission. In 2005 it was estimated that 220,000 children were living with HIV, most of who became infected from their mothers.

Factors contributing to the spread of HIV in Nigeria

Lack of sexual health information and education

Sex is traditionally a very private subject in Nigeria and the discussion of sex with teenagers is often seen as inappropriate. Up until recently there was little or no sexual health education for young people and this has been a major barrier to reducing rates of HIV and other STDs. UNAIDS estimate that only 18 percent of women and 21 percent of men between the ages of 15 and 24 correctly identify ways to prevent HIV. Lack of accurate information about sexual health has meant there are many myths and misconceptions about sex and HIV, contributing to increasing transmission rates as well as stigma and discrimination towards people living with HIV/AIDS.

HIV testing

Another contributing factor to the spread of HIV in Nigeria is the distinct lack of voluntary and routine HIV testing. In a 2003 survey, just 6 percent of women and 14 percent of men had ever been tested for HIV and received the results. In 2005, only around 1 percent of pregnant women were being tested for HIV.

In 2006 president Obasanjo publicly received an HIV test and counseling on World AIDS Day in order to promote the services and information available to people in Nigeria. He stated on the day, "A great majority of Nigerians have now come to accept the reality of AIDS". However, the statistics show that the Nigerian government desperately needs to scale up HIV testing rates in order to bring the epidemic under control.

Cultural practices

Women are particularly affected by the epidemic in Nigeria. In 2006 UNAIDS estimated that women accounted for 61.5 percent of all adults aged 15 and above living with HIV.

Traditionally, women in Nigeria marry young, although the average age at which they marry varies between states. A 2007 study revealed that 54 percent of girls from the North West aged between 15-24 were married by age 15, and 81 percent were married by age 18. The study showed that the younger married girls lacked knowledge on reproductive health, which included HIV/AIDS. They also tend to lack the power and education needed to insist upon the use of a condom during sex. Coupled with the high probability that the husband will be significantly older than the girl and therefore is more likely to have had more sexual partners in the past, young women are more vulnerable to HIV infection within marriage.

Poor healthcare system

Over the last two decades, Nigeria's healthcare system has deteriorated as a result of political instability, corruption and a mismanaged economy. Large parts of the country lack even basic healthcare provision, making it difficult to establish HIV testing and prevention services such as those for the prevention of mother-to-child transmission. Sexual health clinics providing contraception, testing and treatment for other STDs are also few and far between. This makes it particularly difficult to keep the spread of the epidemic under control.

PREVENTION

Condoms

The total number of condoms provided by international donors has been relatively low. One report showed that between 2000 and 2005, the average number of condoms distributed in Nigeria by donors was 5.9 per man, per year[21]. A study in 2002 found that 75 percent of health service facilities that had been visited did not have any condoms or contraceptive supplies.

The number of female condoms sold in Nigeria has significantly increased, which indicates a greater awareness of sexual health issues. In 2003 only 25,000 female condoms had been sold, which increased to 375,000 in 2006. The female condom can potentially help in reducing the spread of HIV, as it does not rely upon the willingness of the man to use a condom himself. However, the female condom is more expensive than the traditional male condom, and is too pricey for the majority of Nigerians.

Restrictions on condom promotion have hampered HIV prevention efforts. In 2001, a radio advertisement was suspended by the Advertising Practitioners Council of Nigeria (APCON) for promoting messages suggesting that it is acceptable to engage in premarital sex as long as a condom is used. In 2006 APCON also started to enforce stricter regulations on condom advertisements that might encourage 'indecency'.

Education

As the majority of new HIV infections occur in young people between the ages of 15 and 25, sex education at school is an important aspect of HIV prevention. In recent years a new curriculum has been introduced for comprehensive sex education for 10-18 year olds. It focuses on improving young people's knowledge and attitudes to sexual health and reducing sexual risk-taking behaviours.

In the past, attempts at providing sex education for young people were hampered by religious and cultural objections. However, the new curriculum was developed with consultation from religious and community leaders and is expected to remain in place in the future.

Media campaigns & public awareness

As Nigeria is such a large and diverse country, media campaigns to raise awareness of HIV are a practical way of reaching many people in different regions. Radio campaigns like the one created by the Society for Family Health are thought to have been successful in increasing knowledge and changing behaviour. "Future Dreams", was a radio serial broadcast in 2001 in nine languages on 42 radio channels. It focused on encouraging consistent condom use, increasing knowledge and increasing skills for condom negotiation in single men and women aged between 18 and 34.

In 2005, a campaign was launched in Nigeria in a bid to raise more public awareness of HIV/AIDS. This campaign took advantage of the recent increase in owners of mobile phones and sent text messages with information about HIV/AIDS to 9 million people.

Another high profile media campaign is fronted by Femi Kuti, the son of Fela Kuti, the famous Afrobeat musician who died of AIDS in 1997. He appears on billboards alongside roads throughout Nigeria with the slogan 'AIDS: No dey show for face', which means you can't tell someone has AIDS by looking at them.

Treatment

When antiretroviral drugs (ARVs) were introduced in Nigeria in the early 1990s, they were only available to those who paid for them. As the cost of the drugs was very high at this time and the overwhelming majority of Nigerians were living on less than $2 a day, only the wealthy minority were able to afford the treatment.

In 2002 the Nigerian government started an ambitious antiretroviral treatment programme, which aimed to supply 10,000 adults and 5,000 children with antiretroviral drugs within one year. An initial $3.5 million worth of ARVs were to be imported from India and delivered at a subsidized monthly cost of $7 per person. The programme was announced as "Africa's largest antiretroviral treatment program".

By 2004 the programme had suffered a major setback as too many patients were being recruited without a big enough supply of drugs to hand out. This resulted in an expanding waiting list and not enough drugs to supply the high demand. The patients who had already started the treatment then had to wait for up to three months for more drugs, which can not only reverse the progress the drugs have already made, but can also increase the risk of HIV becoming resistant to the ARVs. Eventually, another $3.8 million worth of drugs were ordered and the programme resumed.

ARVs were being administered in only 25 treatment centres across the country which was a far from adequate attempt at helping the estimated 550,000 people requiring antiretroviral therapy. As a result, in 2006 Nigeria opened up 41 new AIDS treatment centres and started handing out free ARVs to those who needed them[31].Treatment scale-up between 2006-7 was impressive, rising from 81,000 people (15% of those in need) to 198,000 (26%) by the end of 2007. Despite the progress Nigeria still has a long way to go in providing universal access to anti-AIDS treatment. There are currently 552,000 people in the country who do not have access to the ARV treatment that they need.

The government has set up the National HIV/AIDS Strategic Framework to manage the nation's response from 2005 to 2009. There are a number of targets that have been integrated into the framework. By 2010 Nigeria aims to provide ARVs to 80 percent of adults and children with advanced HIV infection and to 80 percent of HIV-positive pregnant women. The government also aims to test 80 percent of the population for HIV.

These targets could be viewed as over-optimistic, when looking at the situation in Nigeria today. In 2007 only 22 percent of people needing treatment were receiving it. Although this figure has increased from 2.3 percent in 2003, it is still below the average for sub-Saharan Africa.

Funding

It has been estimated that the Nigerian government are contributing around 5 percent of the funds for the antiretroviral treatment programmes. The majority of the funding comes from development partners. The main donors are PEPFAR, the Global Fund and the World Bank.

In 2002, the World Bank loaned US$90.3 million to Nigeria to support the 5-year HIV/AIDS Programme Development Project. In May 2007 it was announced that the World Bank were to allocate a further US$50 million loan for the programme.

From America, PEPFAR (the President's Emergency Plan for AIDS Relief) has allocated a large amount of money to Nigeria. In 2006 PEPFAR gave approximately US$164 million to Nigeria for HIV/AIDS prevention, treatment and care. The planned funding for treatment alone in Nigeria for 2007 was US$138.9, the third highest out of PEPFAR's 15 focus countries.

As of November 2007, the Global Fund has approved nearly US$200 million in funds for Nigeria to expand treatment, prevention, and prevention of mother-to-child transmission programmes. Much of this will be given to the Nigerian government to fund the expansion of antiretroviral treatment.

The future

In the 2007 general elections, Late Umaru Musa Yar'Adua of the People's Democratic Party became the second president of Nigeria's Fourth Republic. Following in

Obasanjo's footsteps, one of Yar'Adua's priorities is tackling the Nigerian HIV/AIDS epidemic.

With the large amounts of money being donated from international funds and a government dedicated to increasing prevention measures and treatment access, some are feeling slightly more optimistic about the future of HIV/AIDS in Nigeria. However, it remains to be seen whether the target of providing universal access to HIV prevention, treatment, care and support by 2010, will be reached.

CHAPTER SIX

HIV AND AIDS IN AFRICA

Sub-Saharan Africa is more heavily affected by HIV and AIDS than any other region of the world. An estimated 22 million people were living with HIV at the end of 2007 and approximately 1.9 million additional people were infected with HIV during that year. In just the past year, the AIDS epidemic in Africa has claimed the lives of an estimated 1.5 million people in this region. More than eleven million children have been orphaned by AIDS.

The extent of the AIDS crisis is only now becoming clear in many African countries, as increasing numbers of people with HIV are becoming ill. In the absence of massively expanded prevention, treatment and care efforts, it is expected that the AIDS death toll in sub-Saharan Africa will continue to rise. This means that impact of the AIDS epidemic on these societies will be felt most strongly in the course of the next ten years and beyond. Its social and economic consequences are already widely felt, not only in the health sector but also in education, industry, agriculture, transport, human resources and the economy in general.

How are different countries in Africa affected?

Both HIV prevalence rates and the numbers of people dying from AIDS vary greatly between African countries. In Somalia and Senegal the HIV prevalence is under 1% of the adult population, whereas in Namibia, South Africa, Zambia and Zimbabwe around 15-20% of adults are infected with HIV.

In three southern African countries, the national adult HIV prevalence rate has risen higher than was thought possible and now exceeds 20%. These countries are Botswana (23.9%), Lesotho (23.2%) and Swaziland (26.1%).

West Africa has been less affected by AIDS, but the HIV prevalence rates in some countries are creeping up. HIV prevalence is estimated to exceed 5% in Cameroon (5.1%) and Gabon (5.9%).

Until recently the national HIV prevalence rate has remained relatively low in Nigeria, the most populous country in sub-Saharan Africa. The rate has grown slowly from below 2% in 1993 to 3.1% in 2007. But some states in Nigeria are already experiencing HIV infection rates as high as those now found in Cameroon. Already around 2.4 million Nigerians are estimated to be living with HIV.

Adult HIV prevalence in East Africa exceeds 5% in Uganda, Kenya and Tanzania.

TRENDS IN AFRICA'S AIDS EPIDEMIC

Large variations exist between the patterns of the AIDS epidemic in different countries in Africa. In some places, the HIV prevalence is still growing. In others the HIV prevalence appears to have stabilised and in a few African nations - such as Kenya and Zimbabwe - declines appear to be under way, probably in part due to effective prevention campaigns. Others countries face a growing danger of explosive growth. The sharp rise in HIV prevalence among pregnant women in Cameroon (more than doubling to over 11% among those aged 20-24 between 1998 and 2000) shows how suddenly the epidemic can surge.

Overall, rates of new HIV infections in sub-Saharan Africa appear to have peaked in the late 1990s, and HIV prevalence seems to have declined slightly, although it remains at an extremely high level. Stabilization of HIV prevalence occurs when the rate of new HIV infections is equaled by the AIDS death rate among the infected population. This means that a country with a stable but very high prevalence must be suffering a very high number of AIDS deaths each year. Although prevalence has declined, the number of Africans living with HIV is rising due to general population growth.

What is the effect of these high levels of HIV infection?

Over and above the personal suffering that accompanies HIV infection, the AIDS epidemic in sub-Saharan Africa threatens to devastate whole communities, rolling back decades of development progress.

Sub-Saharan Africa faces a triple challenge of colossal proportions:

- Providing health care, support and solidarity to a growing population of people with HIV-related illness, and providing them with treatment.
- Reducing the annual toll of new HIV infections by enabling individuals to protect themselves and others.
- Coping with the cumulative impact of over 20 million AIDS deaths on orphans and other survivors, on communities, and on national development.

What is the impact of AIDS on Africa?

HIV & AIDS are having a widespread impact on many parts of African society. The points below describe some of the major effects of the AIDS epidemic.

- In many countries of sub-Saharan Africa, AIDS is erasing decades of progress made in extending life expectancy. Millions of adults are dying from AIDS while they are still young, or in early middle age. Average life expectancy in Sub-Saharan Africa is now 47 years, when it could have been 62 without AIDS.

- The effect of the AIDS epidemic on households can be very severe. Many families are losing their income earners. In other cases, people have to provide AIDS care at home for sick relatives, reducing their capacity to earn money for their family. Many of those dying from AIDS have surviving partners who are themselves infected and in need of care. They leave behind orphans, grieving and struggling to survive without a parent's care.
- In all affected countries, the HIV/AIDS epidemic is putting strain on the health sector. As the epidemic develops, the demand for care for those living with HIV rises, as does the number of health workers affected.
- Schools are heavily affected by HIV/AIDS. This a major concern, because schools can play a vital role in reducing the impact of the epidemic, through education and support.
- HIV/AIDS dramatically affects labour, setting back economic activity and social progress. The vast majority of people living with HIV/AIDS in Africa are between the ages of 15 and 49 - in the prime of their working lives. Employers, schools, factories and hospitals have to train other staff to replace those at the workplace that become too ill to work.

- Through its impacts on the labour force, households and enterprises, HIV/AIDS can act as a significant brake on economic growth and development. HIV/AIDS is already having a major affect on Africa's economic development, and in turn, this affects Africa's ability to cope with the epidemic.

HISTORY OF HIV & AIDS IN AFRICA

AIDS in Africa has had a short but devastating history.

"It all started as a rumour... Then we found we were dealing with a disease.

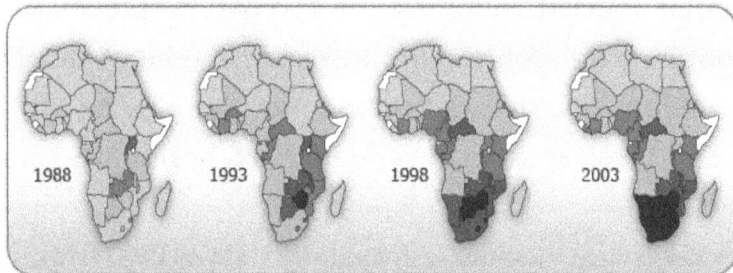

Then we realized that it was an epidemic. And, now we have accepted it as a tragedy." - *Chief epidemiologist in Kampala, Uganda*[1]

ADULT HIV PREVALENCE (%) IN AFRICA BETWEEN 1988 AND 2012

- ▬20%-30%
- ▬10%-20%
- ▬5%-10%
- ▬1%-5%
- ▬0%-1%
- data unavailable

BEFORE THE 1960S – AFRICAN ORIGINS OF AIDS

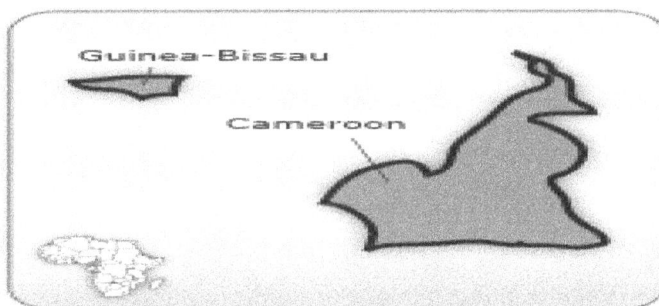

There is now conclusive evidence that HIV originated in Africa. A 10-year study completed in 2012 found a strain of Simian Immunodeficiency Virus (SIV) in a number of chimpanzee colonies in south-east Cameroon that was a viral ancestor of the HIV-1 that causes AIDS in humans. A complex computer model of the evolution of HIV-1 has suggested that the first transfer of SIV to humans occurred around 1930, with HIV-2 transferring from monkeys found in Guinea-Bissau, at some point in the 1940s.

Studies of primates in other continents did not find any trace of SIV, leading to the conclusion that HIV originated in Africa.

THE 1960S- EARLY CASES OF AIDS

Experts studying the spread of the epidemic suggest that about 2,000 people in Africa may have been infected with HIV by the 1960s. Stored blood samples from an American malaria research project carried out in the Congo in 1959 prove one such example of early HIV infection.

THE 1970S – THE FIRST AIDS EPIDEMIC

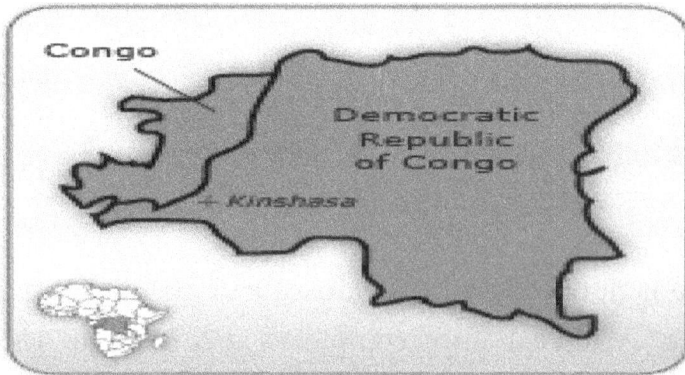

It was in Kinshasa in the 1970s that the first epidemic of HIV/AIDS is believed to have occurred. The emerging epidemic in the Congolese capital was signaled by a surge in opportunistic infections, such as cryptococcal meningitis, Kaposi's sarcoma, tuberculosis and specific forms of pneumonia.

It is speculated that HIV was brought to the city by an infected individual who travelled from Cameroon by river down into the Congo. On arrival in Kinshasa, the virus entered a wide urban sexual network and spread quickly.

The world's first heterosexually-spread HIV epidemic had begun.

THE 1980S – SPREAD AND REACTION

Although HIV was probably carried into Eastern Africa (Uganda, Rwanda, Burundi, Tanzania and Kenya) in the 1970s from its western equatorial origin, it did not reach epidemic levels in the region until the early 1980s.

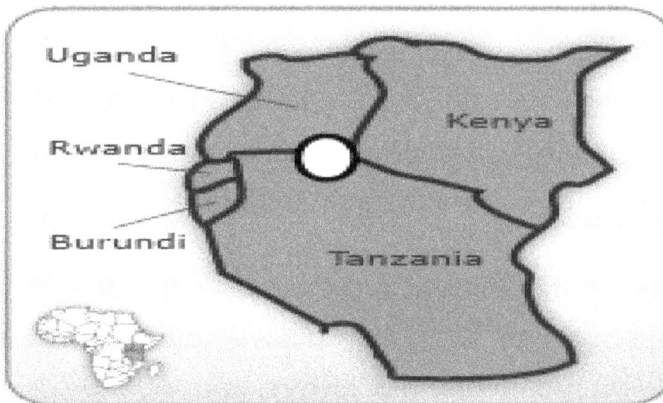

Once HIV was established rapid transmission rates in the eastern region made the epidemic far more devastating than in West Africa, particularly in areas bordering Lake Victoria. The accelerated spread in the region was due to a combination of widespread labour migration, high ratio of men in the urban populations, low status of women, lack of circumcision, and prevalence of sexually transmitted diseases. It is thought that sex workers played a large part in the accelerated transmission rate in East Africa; in Nairobi for example, 85 per cent of sex workers were infected with HIV by 1986.

Uganda was hit very hard by the AIDS epidemic in the 1980s. At the beginning of the decade, doctors were confronted by a surge in cases of a severe wasting disease known locally as 'slim disease', alongside a large number of fatal opportunistic infections such as Kaposi's sarcoma. By this time doctors were aware of AIDS cases with similar symptoms in the United States

> '[b]ut we just could not connect a disease in white, homosexual males in San Francisco to the thing that we were staring at...', David Serwadda, former medical resident at the Uganda Cancer Institute in Kampala.

After the initial clinical recognition of the link between 'slim disease' and AIDS, research was initiated to discover transmission patterns, risk factors, and the prevalence of HIV in Uganda. By the end of the decade HIV prevalence rates amongst pregnant women in Uganda's capital had peaked at over 30 per cent.

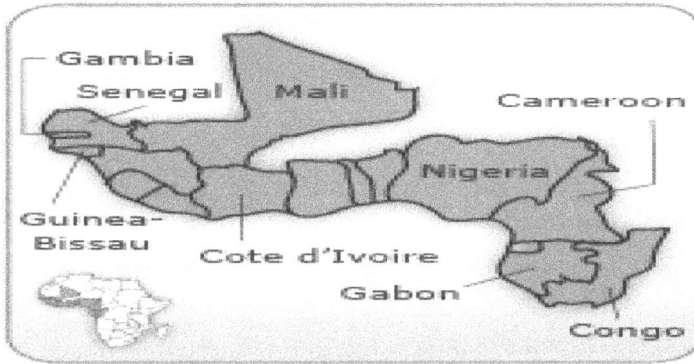

The early 1980s also saw HIV spread further into Western Equatorial Africa and Western African nations. In the Western Equatorial countries of Gabon, Congo-Brazzaville and Cameroon the virus did not cause large epidemics. The long distances between cities, the difficulty of travel, and violence and insecurity meant that there were not the sexual networks that would allow the spread of HIV to epidemic proportions.

West Africa had generally high levels of infection of both HIV-1 and HIV-2, although nowhere near the proportions of East Africa. The HIV-1 epidemic spread across the region beginning with reported cases in Côte d'Ivoire (probably due to rapid urbanization and immigration). By the end of the decade HIV infection had been identified in all of the West African states. Sex work was also a major driver of early infection in West Africa; in Abidjan the former capital of Côte d'Ivoire the HIV prevalence amongst sex workers was already 38% by 1986.

In the mid-1980s the Western African nation of Guinea-Bissau had the world's highest level of HIV-2, with 26% of paid blood donors, 8.6% of pregnant women and 36.7% of sex workers testing positive. The virus spread into rural areas of southern Senegal and The Gambia but HIV-2 was not infectious enough to generate an epidemic beyond this region.

Truck drivers – alongside other migrants such as soldiers, traders and miners - have been identified as a group which facilitated the initial rapid spread of HIV-1 as they engaged with sex workers and spread HIV outwards on the transport and trade routes. In the 1980s, 35 per cent of tested Ugandan truck drivers were HIV positive, as were 30 per cent of military personnel from General Amin's Ugandan army.

In 1988 the second highest prevalence rate of HIV in all of Africa was found on the Tanzam road linking Tanzania and Zambia.

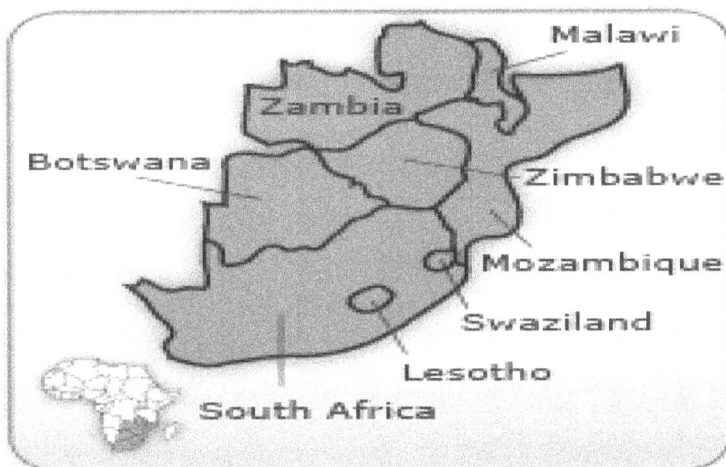

As the decade progressed so too did the epidemic, moving south through Malawi, Zambia, Mozambique, Zimbabwe and Botswana.

Although the virus arrived comparatively late in this region it spurred a devastating epidemic in the general population. By the end of the 1980s the southern African countries of Malawi, Zambia, Zimbabwe and Botswana were on the verge of overtaking East Africa as the focus of the global HIV epidemic.

It is thought that the first case of HIV in South Africa was in a white, homosexual air steward from the USA who died of pneumonia (PCP) in 1982. Blood specimens showed a 16 per cent infection rate among tested gay men in Johannesburg in 1983. The small-scale epidemic was largely confined to white gay men and remained virtually unheard of in the general population in the mid 1980s.

The homosexual epidemic had stopped growing by end of decade[21].

CONFUSION, STIGMA AND DESPONDENCY

The 1980s in Uganda was characterized as a period of *patashika* (confusion) and rumour abounded as to the nature of AIDS. The cause of AIDS was still unclear in the early eighties although it was 'thought to be an infectious agent, probably a virus'. Very little was known about transmission and public anxiety was high. 'They are all simply bewildered' said a Ugandan health worker.

Many questions remained unanswered, most significantly what causes AIDS and how it is transmitted. There were numerous misconceptions, with people thinking that 'you can get HIV through an apple or an orange or an injection or anything' or 'a fat person didn't have HIV' or 'HIV can be transmitted just by looking at a person'. Additionally, confusion with other diseases such as malaria led to overestimations of the transmissibility of HIV and added to the fear surrounding the virus.

Fear quickly bred stigma towards those infected with HIV. Stigma was often related to the association of HIV with prostitution, promiscuity and high-risk lifestyles.

> *"In the early days, when it first came, it was a disease for prostitutes. There were posters with a guy and a bottle of beer and a lady in a*

miniskirt. Those were the ones that were supposed to get HIV".

Because not much was known about HIV/AIDS in the mid-1980s people were often not aware that they were infected with HIV until they had progressed to the final stages of the disease when death was often imminent. This fact coupled with the lack of any effective preventative therapies or treatment meant that there was a reluctance to be tested for the virus.

> *"Why get tested if there was no treatment and no cure – if you were sent home to die, shunned by your family and neighbours".*

GOVERNMENT RESPONSE TO AIDS

With a few notable exceptions the 1980s were characterized by an insufficient response to AIDS in Africa. Often government capacity was saturated by immediate economic concerns, war or political crisis.

As there was no cure or treatment for HIV/AIDS in the 1980s, government strategies had to focus on prevention. Prevention efforts often include encouraging people to revise their sexual behaviour, by abstaining from sex or delaying first sex, being faithful to one partner or having fewer partners, or using condoms consistently and correctly. For this reason prevention efforts in Africa were often confronted with opposition from religious authorities. Both Muslim and Christian leaders found prevention campaigns such as condom promotion difficult to reconcile with their teachings, despite prevailing evidence that abstinence and mutual monogamy were perhaps not as common as they would like.

UNAIDS reported that

> "the fear of offending powerful religious constituencies… created gridlock in some national governments, and for good reason. Conservative lobbies have shown that they can obstruct everything from family life and education to condom promotion if they chose".

Many senior politicians were reluctant to admit to a generalized HIV/AIDS epidemic in their country for fear of creating panic, or discouraging tourism. For this reason it was significant that in 1987 President Kenneth Kaunda of Zambia, a respected African leader, announced to the world that his son, Masuzyo, had died of AIDS.

Uganda and Senegal are often cited as countries that did respond quickly and effectively to the AIDS crisis.

Senegal has one of the lowest rates of HIV in sub-Saharan Africa. The international community often attribute this low prevalence to the prompt response of the government and community organizations to the epidemic, although UNAIDS concedes that it is impossible to predict how the epidemic would have progressed without intervention.

It was not until 1986 when the Ugandan civil war ended and President Museveni was firmly in power that the country got behind a prevention programme. By this time the country was in the midst of a major epidemic, with a prevalence rate of 26% in its capital city.

In 1987 Uganda's AIDS control programme formulated a five-year plan with the assistance of the World Health Organization (WHO). The plan was later made a model for Africa and received more than £20 million in donor funding. The main principles of the campaign were openness and frankness.

Other African nations did not respond to the HIV/AIDS epidemic so positively. In fact, President Mobutu of the Congo banned the subject from the press for four years between 1983 and 1987. Zimbabwean doctors were instructed not to mention AIDS on death certificates, and Côte d'Ivoire, Malawi and Kenya 'ignored the subject entirely or denounced the Western press for 'a new form of hate campaign''.

South Africa's white leaders refused to install an AIDS education programme in schools and did not begin to take seriously the danger of a large-scale heterosexual HIV/AIDS epidemic until the end of the decade.

GLOBAL RESPONSE TO AIDS IN AFRICA

The World Health Organization was slow to respond to the emerging HIV/AIDS epidemic in Africa as it contended that AIDS was not the primary healthcare concern in the region. In 1985 Halfdan Mahler, the Director-General of the organization said "AIDS is not spreading like bush fire in Africa. It is malaria and other tropical diseases that are killing millions of children every day". Realizing quickly the inaccuracy of this statement, the following year Mahler admitted that 'everything is getting worse and worse in AIDS and all of us have been underestimating it, and I in particular'. The WHO Global Programme for the Fight against AIDS was swiftly put into action and aimed to raise $1.5 billion a year by the end of the decade to help prevention and educational efforts[42], with priority to Africa.

In 1987, Jonathon Mann, the director of the Global Programme estimated that one to several million Africans may already have been infected with HIV.

The 1990s – Southern Africa and the Fight for Treatment

The beginning half of the 1990s was a bleak time in the history of AIDS in Africa. At a time when new HIV infection rates were rocketing in Southern Africa there were few new ideas of how to deal with generalized epidemics in poor countries. Prevention campaigns were having minimal effect and there was no visible prospect for effective treatment in Africa. The international community was yet to take efficient action and many national government programmes were corrupt or ill-equipped to deal with the escalating crisis. By the middle of the decade the seriousness of the epidemic was blatant. In 1999, the Kenyan President Daniel Arap Moi declared AIDS a national disaster. "AIDS is not just a serious threat to our social and economic development, it is a real threat to our very existence, and every effort must be made to bring the problem under control".

Although HIV/AIDS prevalence continued to increase in Southern Africa in the later Nineties, glimmers of hope for the future of the epidemic began to emerge.

Prevalence rates in many East African countries that were hard hit in the 1980s were beginning to slow, stabilize or decline. Between 1992 and 1998 prevalence rates in Uganda were estimated to have dropped from 30% to 12% of adults in Kampala. In 1996, UNAIDS was established to take responsibility for coordinating international action against the epidemic.

Rocketing prevalence rates in sub-Saharan Africa

Sub-Saharan Africa was the hub of the HIV epidemic of the 1990s. In 1993 there were an estimated 9 million people infected in the sub-Saharan region out of a global total of 14 million.

In 1998 sub-Saharan Africa was home to 70% of people who became infected with HIV during the year, with an estimated one in seven of these new infections occurring in South Africa.

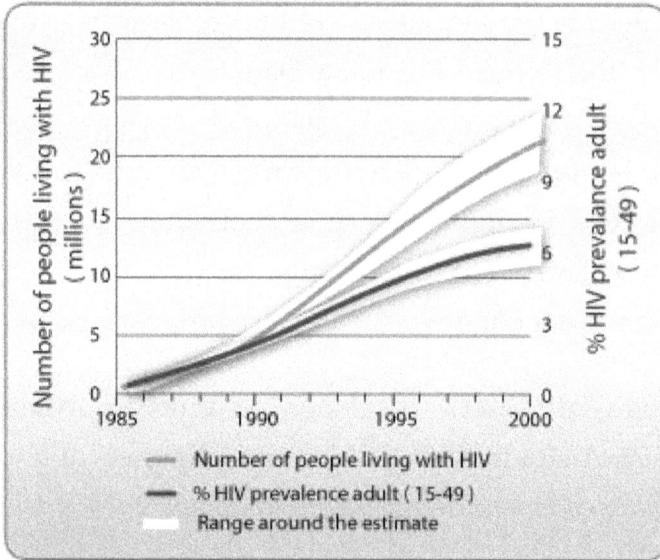

HIV epidemic in Sub-Saharan Africa, 1995-2000.

As HIV/AIDS entered the southern African countries with force, those infected faced high levels of stigma. In 1998, Gugu Dlamini, a South African AIDS activist, was beaten to death by her neighbors after revealing her HIV positive status on Zulu television. This happened just a month after Deputy President Thabo Mbeki had called for people to 'break the silence about AIDS' in order to defeat the epidemic.

South Africa had reacted slowly to the emerging epidemic. The ANC had replaced the apartheid government in 1994 and had concentrated on unifying the country's health systems and expanding primary health care for the poor. This restructuring weakened the health systems just as the HIV/AIDS epidemic was at the peak of expansion. In 1998 the health ministry stopped trials of

AZT to prevent mother-to-child-transmission claiming that it was too expensive and that it would focus its funds on other prevention campaigns. This provoked the first major political action by HIV positive Africans over their own treatment.

The ANC did not work with AIDS organizations and tension between the party and AIDS activists escalated throughout the decade. Due to an increasing frustration with the government's inefficient action against AIDS in 1998 the Treatment Action Campaign (TAC) was founded. Led by Zackie Achmat this group was to become important in the fight for treatment in South Africa.

THE FIGHT FOR TREATMENT

In 1996 the effective combination therapy known as HAART became available for those living with HIV in rich countries. The new drugs were so effective that AIDS death rates in developed countries dropped by 84% over the next four years. This led scientists to declare, 'aggressive treatment with multiple drugs can convert deadly AIDS into a chronic, manageable disorder like diabetes'.

However, as the South African Health Minister, Nkosazana Zuma, pointed out,

> "most people infected with HIV live in Africa,
> where therapies involving combinations of
> expensive antiviral drugs are out of the

question" .

At a cost of $10,000-15,000 per person per year it would cost sub-Saharan countries between 9% and 67% of their GDP to provide triple combination therapy to everybody living with HIV in their countries.

This was clearly impossible for the majority of African nations and the disparity in treatment options angered many people for whom treatment was too expensive. South Africa began to lobby the multi-billion-dollar pharmaceutical corporations of the West to either allow local companies to manufacture HIV/AIDS drugs themselves (this is called compulsory licensing) or import them from other countries, that were producing generic (or copied) drugs at a low cost (this is called parallel importing).

The drug companies argued that if their patents were not protected, there would not be the incentive to do the research and development necessary to continue the fight against AIDS, and they fought vigorously to protect their privileges. The US sided with the pharmaceutical companies and threatened tough sanctions against South Africa.

Eventually, in December 1999 the US and the pharmaceutical companies backed down and Bill Clinton announced that the United States would exercise flexibility in the enforcement of drug patent laws when countries face a public health crisis. The United States approved local production or importation of cheap HIV drugs in South Africa as long as the imported drugs had intellectual property right protection.

This was an initial victory for the fight for treatment in resource poor countries but did not signal an immediate roll out of drugs for those living with AIDS in Africa. For a start not every country had the industry to manufacture drugs locally, or the money to import the drugs, even at a lower cost.

Additionally, this treatment was demanding of clinical services and many governments did not have the healthcare infrastructure to manage large-scale treatment programmes. In the 1980-90s, sub-Saharan Africa had the world's lowest level of social security cover, which includes doctor/patient ratio and access to health services.

In other medical advances in 1994 it was discovered that AZT could reduce mother-to-child-transmission by two-thirds. Although this transformed transmission through pregnancy in developed countries, the cost of about $1,000 per case was prohibitive for those in poor countries. After trials in Thailand showed that a shorter course of AZT also helped to prevent mother-to-child transmission of HIV, the drug company Glaxo Wellcome cut the price of AZT by 75% in 1998. Peter Piot, director of UNAIDS praised the 'hope factor' of the drug and in 1999 Botswana launched Africa's first programme to combat mother to child transmission.

The New Millennium- Global initiatives and drugs roll out

> *"In this effort, there is no us and them, no developed and developing countries, no rich and poor - only a common enemy that knows no frontiers and threatens all people." - Kofi Annan at the G8 summit in Genoa*

Treatment for Africa arrives

In 2000, after mounting pressure to make AIDS drugs more accessible to Africans, five pharmaceutical companies offered to negotiate steep reductions in the prices of AIDS drugs for Africa and other poor regions.

The negotiations were lengthy but over the following few years the world's biggest drug manufacturers frequently cut the price of various patented AIDS drugs until they were only marginally more expensive than the recently approved generic (or 'copied') drugs.

The price reductions were only the first step on the ladder towards universal access to AIDS treatment. Peter Piot, the executive director of UNAIDS said:

> *"This is a promising step in a long-term process... Lowering the price of medicines, however, is only one critical factor in what must become a broader and more urgent effort".*

Practical issues were also of concern. In 2001, the head of USAID Andrew Natsios infamously remarked that:

> *"[Africans] do not know what watches and clocks are. They do not use western means for telling time. They use the sun".*

This comment was in the wider context of western skepticism regarding the feasibility of rolling out antiretroviral treatment to those living with HIV in Africa. The concerns centered on the weak healthcare infrastructure (in 2005 there was a shortage of 1 million professional health workers in Africa) or patients' inability to adhere to treatment (as not taking the drugs at the correct time can lead to drug resistance). The physical delivery of the drugs to remote parts of Africa was also a concern.

In 2001 there were more than 20 [based on current estimates] million people living with AIDS in sub-Saharan Africa, but only 8,000 people in the entire continent were accessing drug treatment.

Joep Lange, the President of the International AIDS Society was optimistic:

> *"If we can get cold Coca Cola and beer to every remote corner of Africa, it should not be impossible to do the same with drugs".*

The debate about the feasibility of providing AIDS drugs to Africa was effectively silenced by the so-called '3 by 5' initiative unveiled by the WHO in 2003. The ambitious programme aimed to put 3 million people in developing countries on antiretrovirals by the end of 2005.

Although the '3 by 5' target was not met, the campaign did manage to substantially increase the number of people on treatment in Africa and raise political support and financial commitment for HIV/AIDS in resource poor countries.

Between 2003 and 2005 the number of people receiving treatment for HIV/AIDS in sub-Saharan Africa increased more than eight-fold to 810 000 from 100 000 people.

At last it seemed that the world was sitting up and taking notice of the ravaging AIDS epidemic in Africa. The amount of money that Western nations were willing to give to help scale-up treatment for those living with AIDS in Africa greatly increased in the new millennium. In 2001, The Global Fund to Fight AIDS, Tuberculosis and Malaria was created and two years later United States President George Bush announced the President's Emergency Plan For AIDS Relief (PEPFAR).

Overall between 2001 and 2004 global funding for AIDS in low-middle income countries trebled to $6.1 billion a year. UNAIDS estimated this to be 50% of all AIDS spending in sub-Saharan Africa during this period. National governments provided 6-10% of funds and the remainder came from families and individuals.

Roll Out

Addressing the UN assembly in June 2001, President Festus Mogae of Botswana voiced his fears of the impact that HIV/AIDS was having on his country.

> *"We are threatened with extinction. People are dying in chillingly high numbers. It is a crisis of the first magnitude."*

The following year Botswana became the first African country to launch a national antiretroviral treatment project. MASA (meaning 'new dawn') was to be equally financed by the Botswana government, the Gates Foundation and the drugs company Merck. Treatment uptake was slow at first as there was a major shortage of health workers and even these few cases overwhelmed the health system. The programme gained momentum and by 2007 approximately 95% of HIV positive people in the country were being treated.

Botswana's successful treatment programme allayed doubts that antiretroviral treatment for poor African countries was unfeasible. It's programme was by far the most successful in Africa, although Namibia (treating 71% of those in need), Rwanda (72%), Kenya (44%), Malawi (43%) Swaziland (42%) Uganda (41%), are also regarded as having being reasonably successful at rolling out treatment.

Less successful were Zimbabwe (impeded by financial and political crisis and lack of trust by global funding bodies), Sudan and Somalia (civil conflict means that data is extremely difficult to collect, estimates lie at around 1% coverage), and Nigeria (due to its extremely weak health system, only 15% of people in need were receiving treatment by 2005).

South Africa's national HIV treatment programme has been the topic of much debate. The South African government was initially hesitant about providing antiretroviral treatment to HIV-positive people, due to unconventional views about HIV and AIDS amongst the government, including President Mbeki's questioning of whether HIV really causes AIDS. After pressure from activists (specifically Treatment Action Campaign TAC) the state began to supply the drugs in 2004. But even since treatment began the distribution of antiretroviral drugs has been relatively slow, with only around 33% of people in need receiving treatment at the end of 2006.

In a decade in which ethical issues were rising up the corporate agenda, a number of large companies also began to provide AIDS treatment programmes for their employees. The vice-president of Anglo American, a large South African mining firm explained that the cost for the firm was justified as the dramatically reduced absenteeism compensated for three-quarters of the cost of the treatment programme.

UNAIDS reported that in total around 17% of those in need of the life-saving drugs in sub-Saharan Africa were receiving them in 2006.

It is increasingly clear that access to drugs to treat HIV/AIDS reduces fear and changes social perceptions of people living with the disease. Antiretrovirals mean that contracting HIV is no longer a death sentence and therefore people are more willing to be tested and find out their HIV status. Although HIV related stigma still exists, it is reducing as fear surrounding the disease lessens and people are more willing to speak openly about AIDS.

As Nelson Mandela said when announcing the death of his son from AIDS in 2005

> *"Let us give publicity to HIV/AIDS and not hide it, because [that is] the only way to make it appear like a normal illness".*

Prevalence and behaviour change

UNAIDS reports that there has been a behavioural change in some parts of Africa in the new millennium. Studies have shown both a substantial increase in condom use since the early 1990's and that younger people have been delaying their sexual début and reducing the number of casual sexual partners.

This trend may account for the reported decline in HIV/AIDS prevalence rates in some parts of Africa, notably Kenya, Zimbabwe and urban areas of Burkina Faso. However, this decline is also likely to be a result of high-mortality rates.

Elsewhere in southern Africa HIV prevalence levels appear to be leveling off (i.e. the number of new infections is roughly matching the number of people who are dying of AIDS) although the stabilization is at very high levels.

AIDS continues to be the leading cause of death in sub-Saharan Africa, in 2007 alone 1.6 million people died of AIDS.

Sixty percent of deaths in sub-Saharan Africa are amongst adults aged between 20 and 49 years. This is causing population imbalances and is removing people at their most economically productive and at a time when they are likely to have young children. An estimated 12 million children in sub-Saharan Africa (which is 9% of the regions children) have lost one or both children to AIDS and this figure is expected to increase as the number of adults dying from AIDS rises over the next decade.

Conclusion

It is estimated that since the beginning of the epidemic more than 15 million Africans have died from AIDS, which is equivalent to the combined populations of London and New York. In this context it becomes possible to understand the massive impact that the AIDS epidemic has had on families, communities, workplaces and national and regional development in Africa.

Although the new millennium has seen a massive increase in global spending to help fight the AIDS epidemic in Africa, there is clearly a long way still to go. Of the 22.5 million people in Africa currently infected with HIV, only 30% of the 7 million people in immediate need of treatment are receiving it.

The recent commitment to universal access to treatment is encouraging but nothing can compensate for the achingly slow regional, national and global response to the AIDS epidemic in Africa. The history of AIDS in Africa is far from complete, not only will the effects of the current epidemic be felt for generations to come, but the lack of a cure for AIDS coupled with limited access to treatment in Africa means that the worst is still not over and millions of people will continue to die.

> *"When this whole thing is over, everyone will stop and cry. But at this point we are numb"* - Winstone Zulu, Zambian AIDS activist

HIV PREVENTION IN AFRICA

A continued rise in the number of Africans living with HIV and dying from AIDS is not inevitable. There is growing evidence that HIV prevention efforts can be effective, and this includes initiatives in some of the most heavily affected countries.

In some countries there have been early and sustained HIV prevention efforts. For example, effective HIV prevention campaigns have been carried out in Senegal, which is still reflected in the relatively low adult HIV prevalence rate of 0.9%. Also, the experience of Uganda shows that a widespread AIDS epidemic can be brought under control. HIV prevalence in Uganda fell from around 15% in the early 1990s to around 5% by 2001. This change is thought to be largely due to intensive HIV prevention campaigns.

More recently, similar declines have been seen in Kenya, Zimbabwe and urban areas of Zambia and Burkina Faso. However, the extremely severe AIDS epidemics in South Africa, Swaziland and Mozambique continue to grow.

Overall a massive expansion in prevention efforts is needed, and although there is no single or immediate tool to prevent new HIV infections, the major components of a successful HIV prevention programme are now known.

Condom use & HIV

Condoms play a key role in preventing HIV infection around the world. In Sub-Saharan Africa, most countries have seen an increase in condom use in recent years. In studies carried out between 2001 and 2005, eight out of eleven countries in sub-Saharan Africa reported an increase in condom use.

The distribution of condoms to countries in sub-Saharan Africa has also increased: in 2004 the number of condoms provided to this region by donors was equivalent to 10 for every man, compared to 4.6 for every man in 2001. In most countries, though, many more condoms are still needed. For instance, in Uganda between 120 and 150 million condoms are required annually, but less than 40 million were provided in 2005.

Relative to the enormity of the HIV/AIDS epidemic in Africa, providing condoms is cheap and cost effective. Even when condoms are available, though, there are still a number of social, cultural and practical factors that may prevent people from using them. In the context of stable partnerships where pregnancy is desired, or where it may be difficult for one partner to suddenly suggest condom use, this option may not be practical.

Provision of HIV Counseling & Testing (HCT)

The provision of HIV counseling and testing (HCT) is an important part of any national prevention program. It is widely recognized that individuals living with HIV who are aware of their status are less likely to transmit HIV infection to others, and that through testing they can be directed to care and support that can help them to stay healthy. VCT also provides benefit for those who test negative, in that their behaviour may change as a result of the test.

The provision of VCT has become easier, cheaper and more effective as a result of the introduction of rapid HIV testing, which allows individuals to be tested and find out the results on the same day. VCT could – and indeed needs to be – made more widely available in most sub-Saharan African countries.

Mother-to-child transmission of HIV

Around 2 million children in sub-Saharan Africa were living with HIV at the end of 2007. They represent more than 85% of all children living with HIV worldwide. The vast majority of these children will have become infected with HIV during pregnancy or through breastfeeding when they are babies, as a result of their mother being HIV-positive.

Mother to child transmission (MTCT) of HIV is not inevitable. Without interventions, there is a 20-45% chance that a HIV-positive mother will pass infection on to her child. If a woman is supplied with antiretroviral drugs, though, this risk can be reduced significantly. Before this measures can be taken the mother must be aware of her HIV-positive status, so testing also plays a vital role in the prevention of MTCT.

In many developed countries, these steps have helped to virtually eliminate MTCT. Yet Sub-Saharan Africa continues to be severely affected by the problem, due to a lack of drugs, services and information. The shortage of testing facilities in many areas is also contributing. In 2006, preventive drugs reached only 31% of HIV-infected pregnant women in Eastern and Southern Africa, and only 7% in West and Central Africa.

Given the scale of the MTCT crisis in Africa, it is remarkable that more is not being done (by both the international community and domestic governments) to prevent the rising numbers of children becoming infected with HIV, and dying from AIDS. I am calling for vast improvements in preventing MTCT strategies through our Stop AIDS in Children campaign.

HIV/AIDS RELATED TREATMENT AND CARE IN AFRICA

Antiretroviral drugs

Antiretroviral drugs (ARVs) - which significantly delay the progression of HIV to AIDS and allow people living with HIV to live relatively normal, healthy lives – have been available in richer parts of the world since around 1996. Distributing these drugs requires money, a well-structured health system and a sufficient supply of healthcare workers. The majority of developing countries is lacking in these areas and has struggled to cope with the increasing numbers of people requiring treatment.

For most Africans living with HIV, ARVs are still not available - fewer than one in five of the millions of Africans in need of the treatment are receiving it. Many millions are not even receiving treatment for opportunistic infections, which affect individuals whose immune systems have been weakened by HIV infection. These facts reflect the world's continuing failure, despite the progress of recent years, to mount a response that matches the scale and severity of the global HIV/AIDS epidemic.

Botswana pioneered the provision of ARVs in Africa, starting its national treatment programme in January 2002. By 2005 this programme was providing treatment to the vast majority of those in need. According to World Health Organization figures, 93,000 people were receiving treatment at the end of 2007, including those using the private sector, giving a coverage rate of around 80%. Thousands of lives have been saved as a result.

While most African countries have now started to distribute ARVs, progress in providing sufficient quantities of the drugs has been uneven and Botswana's success has not been emulated elsewhere. Among the other countries that have made advances are Rwanda and

Namibia, where more than 70% of people in need of ARVs are receiving them. In Cameroon, Côte d'Ivoire, Kenya, Malawi and Nigeria, between 25% and 45% of people requiring antiretroviral drugs were receiving them in December 2007. While South Africa is the richest nation in Sub-Saharan Africa and should have led the way in ARV distribution, its government was slow to act; so far, only 28% of those in need of treatment in South Africa are receiving it. In other countries, such as Chad, Congo, Ghana, Sudan and Zimbabwe, the figure is less than 20%.

Nonetheless, the overall situation is slowly improving; the number of people receiving ARVs in Africa doubled in 2005 alone. International support has helped this increase, with numerous governments and international organizations encouraging progress. In 2003 the World Health Organization (WHO) initiated the '3 by 5' programme, which aimed to have three million people in developing countries on ARVs by the end of 2005. While this target was not reached, a number of African nations made substantial progress under the scheme. The latest international target, 'All by 2010', is aiming at universal access to treatment by 2010. In pursuit of this goal it is hoped that considerable progress will be made in Africa's fight against AIDS. There are still, however, a number of impediments to ARV provision. One major challenge is the fact that the majority of African countries have a poor healthcare infrastructure and a shortage of medical professionals. A considerable emphasis needs to place not only on the availability of ARVs, but also the availability of professionals who are able to administer the drugs.

Another major challenge is ensuring that drugs are not only supplied to a lot of areas, but that *sufficient quantities* of drugs are supplied to those areas. This is critically important; because once an individual starts to take ARVs they have to take them for the rest of their life. If, for instance, their local hospital runs out of ARVs, the interruption that this causes in their treatment could result in them becoming resistant to the drugs. To improving treatment programs, African countries face the double challenge of getting new people to start treatment and maintaining the supply of treatment to those who are already receiving ARVs.

Other forms of treatment and care

Treatment and care for HIV consists of a number of different elements apart from ARVs. These include voluntary counseling and testing, food and management of nutritional effects, follow-up counseling, protection from stigma and discrimination, treatment of other sexually transmitted infections, and the prevention and treatment of opportunistic infections. All of these things can, and indeed should, be provided before ARVs are available. This does not exclude the provision of ARVs when they are available. Indeed, when ARVs do become available the provision of antiretroviral therapy should be easier and quicker to implement because many of the things apart from drugs that are needed for successful treatment are already in place.

CHAPTER SEVEN

MAKING A DIFFERENCE IN AFRICA

International support

One of the most important ways in which the situation in Africa can be improved is through increased funding for HIV/AIDS. More money would help to improve both prevention campaigns and the provision of treatment and care for those living with HIV. Developed countries have increased funding for the fight against AIDS in Africa in recent years, perhaps most significantly through the Global Fund to fight AIDS, Tuberculosis and Malaria. The Global Fund was started in 2001 to co-ordinate international funding and has since approved grants totaling US $3.3 billion to fight HIV and AIDS in Africa. Around 60% of the fund's grants have been directed towards Africa and 60% has been put towards fighting AIDS.[12] This funding is making a significant difference, but given the massive scale of the AIDS epidemic more money is still needed.

The US Government has shown a commitment to fighting AIDS in Africa through the President's Emergency Plan For AIDS Relief (PEPFAR). Started in 2003, PEPFAR provides money to fight AIDS in numerous countries, including 15 focus countries, most of which are African. In Fiscal Year 2005, PEPFAR allocated US $1.1 billion to these African focus countries. The US Government is also the largest contributor to the Global Fund.

Among other things, organizations like PEPFAR and the Global Fund provide vital support to local and community groups that are working 'on the ground' to provide relief in Africa. These groups are directly helping people in need, and many rely on international funding in order to operate. Getting money from large, international donors to small, 'grassroots organizations can present a number of difficulties though, as money is lost or delayed as it is passed down large funding chains.

Domestic commitment

More than money is needed if HIV prevention and treatment programmes are to be scaled up in Africa. In order to implement such programmes, a country's health, education, communications and other infrastructures must be sufficiently developed. In some African countries these systems are already under strain and are at risk of collapsing as a result of AIDS. Money can also only be used efficiently if there are sufficient human resources available, but there is an acute shortage of trained personnel in many parts of Africa.

In many cases, African countries also need more commitment from their governments. There are promising signs that some governments are starting to respond and becoming more involved in the fight against

AIDS, and this commitment needs to be sustained if the severe impact of Africa's AIDS pandemic is to be reduced.

Reducing stigma and discrimination

HIV-related stigma and discrimination remains an enormous barrier to the fight against AIDS. Fear of discrimination often prevents people from getting tested, seeking treatment and admitting their HIV status publicly. Since laws and policies alone cannot reverse the stigma that surrounds HIV infection, more and better AIDS education is needed in Africa to combat the ignorance that causes people to discriminate. The fear and prejudice that lies at the core of HIV/AIDS discrimination needs to be tackled at both community and national levels.

Helping women and girls

In many parts of Africa, as elsewhere in the world, the AIDS epidemic is aggravated by social and economic inequalities between men and women. Women and girls commonly face discrimination in terms of access to education, employment, credit, health care, land and inheritance. These factors can all put women in a position where they are particularly vulnerable to HIV infection. In sub-Saharan Africa, around 59% of those living with HIV are female.

In many African countries, sexual relationships are dominated by men, meaning that women cannot always practice safe sex even when they know the risks involved. Attempts are currently being made to develop a microbicide – a cream or gel that can be applied to the vagina, preventing HIV infection – which could be a significant breakthrough in protecting women against HIV. Women could apply such a microbicide without their partner even knowing. It is likely to be some time before a microbicide is ready for use, though, and even when it is, women will only use it if they have an awareness and understanding of HIV and AIDS. To promote this, a greater emphasis needs to be placed on educating women and girls about AIDS, and adapting education systems (which are currently male-dominated) to their needs.

The way forward

Tackling the AIDS crisis in Africa is a long-term task that requires sustained effort and planning - both within African countries themselves and amongst the international community. One of the most important elements of the fight against AIDS is the prevention of new HIV infections. HIV prevention campaigns that have been successful within African countries need to be highlighted and repeated.

The other main challenge is providing treatment and care to those living with HIV in Africa, in particular ARVs, which can allow people living with HIV to live long and healthy lives. Many African countries have made significant progress in their treatment programmes in recent years and it is likely that the next few years will see many more people receiving the drugs.

The impact of HIV & AIDS in Africa

Two-thirds of all people living with HIV are found in sub-Saharan Africa, although this region contains little more than 10% of the world's population.[1] AIDS has caused immense human suffering in the continent. The most obvious effect of this crisis has been illness and death, but the impact of the epidemic has certainly not been confined to the health sector; households, schools, workplaces and economies have also been badly affected.

During 2007 alone, an estimated 1.5 million adults and children died as a result of AIDS in sub-Saharan Africa. Since the beginning of the epidemic more than 15 million Africans have died from AIDS.

Although antiretroviral treatment is starting to lessen the toll of AIDS, still fewer than one in three Africans who need treatment are receiving it. The impact of AIDS will remain severe for many years to come.

The Impact on the Health Sector

In all affected countries the AIDS epidemic is bringing additional pressure to bear on the health sector. As the epidemic matures, the demand for care for those living with HIV rises, as does the toll of AIDS on health workers.

In sub-Saharan Africa, the direct medical costs of AIDS (excluding antiretroviral therapy) have been estimated at about US$30 per year for every person infected, at a time when overall public health spending is less than US$10 per year for most African countries.

The Effect on Hospitals

As the HIV prevalence of a country rises, the strain placed on its hospitals is likely to increase. In sub-Saharan Africa, people with HIV-related diseases occupy more than half of all hospital beds. Government-funded research in South Africa has suggested that, on average, HIV-positive patients stay in hospital four times longer than other patients.

Hospitals are struggling to cope, especially in poorer African countries where there are often too few beds available. This shortage results in people being admitted only in the later stages of illness, reducing their chances of recovery.

Health Care Workers

While AIDS is causing an increased demand for health services, large numbers of healthcare professionals are being directly affected by the epidemic. Botswana, for example, lost 17% of its healthcare workforce due to AIDS between 1999 and 2005. A study in one region of Zambia found that 40% of midwives were HIV-positive. Healthcare workers are already scarce in most African countries. Excessive workloads, poor pay and migration to richer countries are among the factors contributing to this shortage.

Although the recent increase in the provision of antiretroviral drugs (which significantly delay the progression from HIV to AIDS) has brought hope to many in Africa, it has also put increased strain on healthcare workers. Providing antiretroviral treatment to everyone who needs it requires more time and training than is currently available in most countries.

The Impact on Households

The toll of HIV and AIDS on households can be very severe. Although no part of the population is unaffected by HIV, it is often the poorest sectors of society that are most vulnerable to the epidemic and for whom the consequences are most severe. In many cases, the presence of AIDS causes the household to dissolve, as parents die and children are sent to relatives for care and upbringing. A study in rural South Africa suggested that households in which an adult had died from AIDS were four times more likely to dissolve than those in which no deaths had occurred. Much happens before this dissolution takes place: AIDS strips families of their assets and income earners, further impoverishing the poor.

Household Income

In Botswana it is estimated that, on average, every income earner is likely to acquire one additional dependent over the next ten years due to the AIDS epidemic. A dramatic increase in destitute households – those with no income earners – is also expected. Other countries in the region are experiencing the same problem, as individuals who would otherwise provide a household with income are prevented from working by HIV and AIDS – either because they are ill themselves or because they are caring for another sick family member.

Such a situation is likely to have repercussions for every member of the family. Children may be forced to abandon their education and in some cases women may be forced to turn to sex work ('prostitution'). This can lead to a higher risk of HIV transmission, which further exacerbates the situation.

Basic Necessities

A study in South Africa found that already poor households coping with members who are sick from HIV or AIDS were reducing spending on necessities even further. The most likely expenses to be cut were clothing (21%), electricity (16%) and other services (9%). Falling incomes forced about 6% of households to reduce the amount they spent on food and almost half of households reported having insufficient food at times.

"She then led me to the kitchen and showed me empty buckets of food and said they had nothing to eat that day just like other days."

Food Production

The AIDS epidemic adds to food insecurity in many areas, as agricultural work is neglected or abandoned due to household illness. In Malawi, where food shortages have had a devastating effect, it has been recognized that HIV and AIDS are diminishing the country's agricultural output. It is thought that by 2020, Malawi's agricultural workforce will be 14% smaller than it would have been without HIV and AIDS. In other countries, such as Mozambique, Botswana, Namibia and Zimbabwe, the reduction is likely to be over 20%.

A recent study in Kenya demonstrated that food production in households in which the head of the family died of AIDS were affected in different ways depending on the sex of the deceased. As in other sub-Saharan African countries, it was generally found that the death of a male reduced the production of 'cash crops' (such as coffee, tea and sugar), while the death of a female reduced the production of grain and other crops necessary for household survival.

Healthcare expenses and funeral costs

Taking care of a person sick with AIDS is not only an emotional strain for household members, but also a major strain on household resources. Loss of income, additional care-related expenses, the reduced ability of caregivers to work, and mounting medical fees push affected households deeper into poverty. It is estimated that, on average, HIV-related care can absorb one-third of a household's monthly income.

The financial burden of death can also be considerable, with some families in South Africa easily spending seven times their total household monthly income on a funeral. Furthermore, although many South Africans contribute to some sort of funeral insurance plan, many of these are inadequately funded, and it is arguable that such financial arrangements detract from other savings plans or health insurance.

Aside from the financial burden, providing AIDS care at home can impose demands on the physical, mental and general health of carers – usually family and friends of the sick person. Such risks are amplified if carers are untrained or unsupported by a home-based care organisation.

How do HIV/AIDS affected households cope in Africa?

Three main coping strategies appear to be adopted among affected households. Savings are used up or assets sold; assistance is received from other households; and the composition of households tends to change, with fewer adults of prime working age in the households.

Almost invariably, the burden of coping rests with women. Upon a family member becoming ill, the role of women as carers, income-earners and housekeepers is stepped up. They are often forced to step into roles outside their homes as well. In parts of Zimbabwe, for example, women are moving into the traditionally male-dominated carpentry industry. This often results in women having less time to prepare food and for other tasks at home.

> *"I used to stay with the children, but now it is a problem. I have to work in the fields. Last year I had more money to hire labour so the crops got weeded more often. This year I had to do it myself."* Angelina, Zimbabwe

Older people are also heavily affected by the epidemic; many have to care for their sick children and are often left to look after orphaned grandchildren. AVERT has more about how older people are affected by the HIV/AIDS epidemic.

Tapping into savings if available and taking on more debt are usually the first options chosen by households struggling to pay for medical treatment or funerals. Then as debts mount, precious assets such as bicycles, livestock and even land are sold. Once households are stripped of their productive assets, the chances of them recovering and rebuilding their livelihoods become even slimmer.

The number of working adults in a family will often decrease.

> *"Our fields are idle because there is nobody to work them. We don't have machinery for farming, we only have manpower - if we are sick, or spend our time looking after family members who are sick, we have no time to spend working in the fields."* Toby Solomon, commissioner for the Nsanje district, Malawi

One of the more unfortunate responses to a death in poorer households is removing the children (especially girls) from school. Often the school uniforms and fees become unaffordable for the families and the child's labour and income-generating potential are required in the household.

> *"Because I'm a poor African woman, I can't raise enough money for three orphans. The one in secondary school, sometimes she misses first term because I'm looking for tuition. The others miss schools for two or three days at a time. I had a cow I used to milk, but as time went on the cow died, so I can't find any other income…"* Barbara, Uganda

The Impact on Children

It is hard to overemphasize the trauma and hardship that children affected by HIV and AIDS are forced to bear. The epidemic not only causes children to lose their parents or guardians, but sometimes their childhood as well.

As parents and family members become ill, children take on more responsibility to earn an income, produce food and care for family members. It is harder for these children to access adequate nutrition, basic health care, housing and clothing. Fewer families have the money to send their children to school.

Often both of the parents are HIV positive in Africa. Consequently, more children have been orphaned by AIDS in Africa than anywhere else. Many children are now raised by their grandparents or left on their own in child-headed households.

As projections of the number of AIDS orphans rise, some have called for an increase in institutional care for children. However this solution is not only expensive but also detrimental to the children. Institutionalization stores up problems for society, which is ill equipped to cope with an influx of young adults who have not been socialized in the community in which they have to live. There are other alternatives available. One example is the approach developed by church groups in Zimbabwe, in which community members are recruited to visit orphans in their homes, where they live either with foster parents, grandparents or other relatives, or in child-headed households.

The way forward is prevention. Firstly, it is crucial to prevent children from becoming infected with HIV at birth as well as later in life. Secondly, if efforts are made to prevent adults becoming infected with HIV, and to care for those already infected, then fewer children will be orphaned by AIDS in the future.

The Impact on the Education Sector

The relationship between AIDS and the education sector is circular – as the epidemic worsens, the education sector is damaged, which in turn is likely to increase the incidence of HIV transmission. There are numerous ways in which AIDS can affect education, but equally there are many ways in which education can help the fight against AIDS. The extent to which schools and other education institutions are able to continue functioning will influence how well societies eventually recover from the epidemic.

> *"Without education, AIDS will continue its rampant spread. With AIDS out of control, education will be out of reach."*

Peter Piot, Director of UNAIDS[20]

Fewer Children Receiving a Basic Education

A decline in school enrolment is one of the most visible effects of the epidemic. This in itself will have an effect on HIV prevention, as a good basic education ranks among the most effective and cost-effective means of preventing HIV.

There are numerous barriers to school attendance in Africa. Children may be removed from school to care for parents or family members, or they may themselves be living with HIV. Many are unable to afford school fees and other such expenses – this is particularly a problem among children who have lost their parents to AIDS, who often struggle to generate income.

Studies have suggested that young people with little or no education may be 2.2 times more likely to contract HIV as those who have completed primary education.[22] In this context, the devastating effect that AIDS is having on school enrolment is a big concern. In Swaziland and the Central African Republic, it has been reported that school enrolment has fallen by 25-30% due to AIDS.

The Impact on Teachers

HIV/AIDS affects teachers as well as pupils. In the early stages of the African epidemic it was reported that teachers were at a higher risk of becoming infected with HIV than the general population, because of their relatively high socio-economic status and a lack of understanding about how the virus is transmitted. This trend appears to have changed, as evidence increasingly shows that the more educated an individual is, the more likely they are to change their behaviour.[24] But HIV and

AIDS are still having a devastating affect on the already inadequate supply of teachers in African countries; for example, a study in South Africa found that 21% of teachers aged 25-34 are living with HIV.

Teachers who are affected by HIV and AIDS are likely to take increasing periods of time off work. Those with sick families may also take time off to attend funerals or to care for sick or dying relatives, and further absenteeism may result from the psychological effects of the epidemic.

When a teacher falls ill, the class may be taken on by another teacher, may be combined with another class, or may be left untaught. Even when there is a sufficient supply of teachers to replace losses, there can be a significant impact on the students. This is particularly concerning given the important role that teachers can play in the fight against AIDS. One example is the benefits that a good teacher can give to children who have lost their parents to AIDS:

> *"It is important to recognize teachers as key partners in the care of orphans and vulnerable children. A teacher's attitude can do much towards acceptance, or rejection and stigmatization, of an orphan in a classroom. Teachers need to be trained in recognizing the behavioral problems associated with unsolved grief."* Dr Sue Perry, Zimbabwe.

The illness or death of teachers is especially devastating in rural areas where schools depend heavily on one or two teachers. Moreover, skilled teachers are not easily replaced. Tanzania has estimated that it needs around 45,000 additional teachers to make up for those who have died or left work because of HIV and AIDS. The greatest proportion of staff that have been lost, according to the Tanzania Teacher's Union, were experienced staff between the ages of 41 and 50.

The Impact on Enterprises and Workplaces

HIV and AIDS dramatically affect labour, setting back economic and social progress. The vast majority of people living with HIV in Africa are between the ages of 15 and 49 - in the prime of their working lives.

AIDS damages businesses by squeezing productivity, adding costs, diverting productive resources, and depleting skills. Company costs for health-care, funeral benefits and pension fund commitments are likely to rise as the number of people taking early retirement or dying increases. Also, as the impact of the epidemic on households grows more severe, market demand for products and services can fall. The epidemic hits productivity through increased absenteeism. Comparative studies of East African businesses have shown that absenteeism can account for as much as 25-54% of company costs.

A study in several Southern African countries has estimated that the combined impact of AIDS-related absenteeism, productivity declines, health-care expenditures, and recruitment and training expenses could cut profits by at least 6-8%.[30] Another study of a thousand companies in Southern Africa found that 9% had suffered a significant negative impact due to AIDS. In areas that have been hit hardest by the epidemic, it found that up to 40% of companies reported that HIV and AIDS were having a negative effect on profits.

Some companies, though, have implemented successful programs to deal with the epidemic. An example is the gold-mining industry in South Africa. The gold mines attract thousands of workers, often from poor and remote regions. Most live in hostels, separated from their families; as a result a thriving sex industry operates around many mines and HIV is common. In recent years, mining companies have been working with a number of organizations to implement prevention programmes for the miners. These have included mass distribution of condoms, medical care and treatment for sexually transmitted diseases, and awareness campaigns. Some mining companies have started to replace all-male hostels with accommodation for families, in order to reduce the transmission of HIV and other sexually transmitted diseases.

In Swaziland, an employers' anti-AIDS coalition has been set up to promote voluntary counseling and testing. The coalition not only includes larger companies but also small and medium sized enterprises. In Botswana, the Debswana diamond company offers all employees HIV testing, and provides antiretroviral drugs to HIV positive workers and their spouses. This policy was introduced in 1999 when the company found that many of their workforce were HIV positive. With a skilled workforce, it is financially worth their while to protect the health and therefore the productivity of their workers. Nevertheless, workplace programmes for HIV treatment and prevention remain scarce in Africa.

The Impact on Life Expectancy

In many countries of sub-Saharan Africa, AIDS is erasing decades of progress in extending life expectancy. In the worst affected countries, average life expectancy has fallen by twenty years because of the epidemic. Life expectancy at birth in Swaziland is just 31 years - less than half of what it would be without AIDS.

The impact that AIDS has had on average life expectancy is partly attributed to child mortality, as increasing numbers of babies are born with HIV infections acquired from their mothers. The biggest increase in deaths, however, has been among adults aged between 20 and 49 years. This group now accounts for 60% of all deaths in sub-Saharan Africa, compared to 20% between 1985 and 1990, when the epidemic was in its early stages. By affecting this age group so heavily, AIDS is hitting adults in their most economically productive years and removing the very people who could be responding to the crisis.

The Economic Impact

Through its impacts on the labour force, households and enterprises, AIDS has played a more significant role in the reversal of human development than any other single factor. One aspect of this development reversal has been the damage that the epidemic has done to the economy, which, in turn, has made it more difficult for countries to respond to the crisis. One way in which HIV and AIDS affect the economy is by reducing the labour supply through increased mortality and illness. Amongst those who are able to work, productivity is likely to decline as a result of HIV-related illness. Government income also declines, as tax revenues fall and governments are pressured to increase their spending to deal with the expanding HIV epidemic.

The abilities of African countries to diversify their industrial base, expand exports and attract foreign investment are integral to economic progress in the region. By making labour more expensive and reducing profits, AIDS limits the ability of African countries to attract industries that depend on low-cost labour and makes investments in African businesses less desirable. HIV and AIDS therefore threaten the foundations of economic development in Africa.

The impact that AIDS has had on the economies of African countries is difficult to measure. The economies of the worst affected countries were already struggling with development challenges, debt and declining trade before the epidemic started to affect the continent. AIDS has combined with these factors to further aggravate the situation. It is thought that the impact of AIDS on the gross domestic product (GDP) of the worst affected countries is a loss of around 1.5% per year; this means that after 25 years the economy would be 31% smaller than it would otherwise have been. One way in which this impact can be reduced is through the provision of antiretroviral drugs to people living with HIV. A study in South Africa suggested that if ARV coverage expanded to reach 50% of those in need of the drugs then the effect of the epidemic on economic growth would be reduced by 17%.

CHAPTER EIGHT

THE FUTURE IMPACT OF HIV/AIDS

This page has outlined just some of the ways in which the AIDS epidemic has had a significant impact on countries in sub-Saharan Africa. Although both international and domestic efforts to overcome the crisis have been strengthened in recent years, there is little sign of the epidemic diminishing. The people of sub-Saharan Africa will continue to feel the effects of HIV and AIDS for many years to come. It is clear that as much as possible needs to be done to minimise this impact.

As access to treatment is slowly expanded throughout the continent, millions of lives are being extended and hope is being given to people who previously had none. Unfortunately though, the majority of people in need of treatment are still not receiving it, and campaigns to prevent new infections (which must remain the central focus of the fight against AIDS) are lacking in many areas.

AIDS in Africa is linked to many other problems, such as poverty and poor public infrastructures. Efforts to fight the epidemic must take these realities into account, and look at ways in which the general development of Africa can progress. As the evidence discussed in this page makes clear, however, AIDS is acting as the single greatest barrier to Africa's development. Much wider access to HIV prevention, treatment and care services is urgently needed.

Timeline of AIDS in Africa

This timeline features some of the most important developments in the history of AIDS in Africa. Much more detailed information an be found in our individual Africa country pages.

Events are divided into five categories as follows:

- Spread of AIDS
- Science and prevention
- Treatment
- Global action
- National event

Before 1970s

- A form of simian immunodeficiency virus probably transfers to humans in Central Africa around 1930. The mutated virus would later become known as HIV-1.
- The virus that would later become known as HIV-2 probably transfers to humans from sooty mangabey monkeys in Guinea-Bissau, West Africa around 1960.

1970s

- Doctors in Zaire (later DRC) and Burundi see a rise in certain infections such as cryptococcal meningitis and PCP, a type of pneumonia, as well as diarrhoea and severe wasting.

1982

- A fatal wasting disease, known locally as 'slim', is becoming increasingly common in South West Uganda.

1983

- Heterosexually transmitted AIDS is noticed in a group of African patients in Belgium.
- Doctors in Zambia and Zaire are aware of a new aggressive form of Kaposi's sarcoma, which had previously been endemic but non-fatal.

1984

- Western scientists confirm that AIDS is widespread in parts of Africa, with strong indications of heterosexual transmission.
- The first AIDS research project in Africa, 'Project SIDA' is launched in Kinshasa, DRC.

1985

- Western scientists debate whether "slim disease" in Uganda is a new syndrome or identical to AIDS.

1986

- Uganda begins promoting sexual behaviour change in response to AIDS.

1987

- The first antiretroviral drug (AZT) is licensed to treat people with HIV, but is unavailable to virtually everyone in Africa.
- President Kaunda of Zambia announces that his son has died of AIDS.
- There have been 2,369 reported AIDS cases in Uganda and 1,608 in Tanzania.
- The AIDS Support Organization (TASO) is founded in Uganda.

1990

- There are an estimated 5,500,000 HIV cases in Africa and more than 650,000 estimated AIDS cases.

1993

- An estimated 9 million adults in sub-Saharan Africa are infected with HIV, with 1.7 million AIDS cases.
- The recorded number of HIV infections in South Africa grows by 60% in two years.

1995

- There are an estimated 1.9 million new infections in sub-Saharan Africa.

1996

- HIV prevalence among young pregnant women in Lesotho shoots up to 26% from 3.9% in 1992.
- Effective combination therapy drugs become widely available in the West but are too expensive for most people living with AIDS in Africa.

1997

- Fela Kuti, Nigeria's most famous musician dies of Kaposi's Sarcoma, an AIDS-related illness.

1998

- A South African AIDS activist, Gugu Dlamini, is beaten to death by her neighbours after revealing her HIV positive status on television.

- HIV infections in sub-Saharan Africa account for 70% of infections worldwide.
- The Treatment Action Campaign (TAC) is founded by Zackie Achmat to lobby the South African government for access to AIDS drugs.

1999

- The South African President, Thabo Mbeki, disputes the efficacy of Western AIDS drugs, claiming that AZT is toxic.
- Nevirapine, a new single dose drug, provides hope for the future prevention of mother-to-child-transmission of HIV in Africa.

2000

- Two thirds of 15 year-old children in Botswana are predicted to die of AIDS before they reach 50.
- Five pharmaceutical companies offer to negotiate steep reductions in the prices of AIDS drugs for Africa.
- An International AIDS Conference is held in Africa for the first time.
- President Mbeki withdraws from the "does HIV cause AIDS" debate after causing much controversy.

2001

- It is estimated that 4.7 million South Africans are HIV-positive, including 24.5% of pregnant women.
- There are 1 million AIDS orphans in Zimbabwe.
- Nkosi Johnson, who famously fought for the rights of HIV positive people in South Africa, dies of AIDS aged twelve.

2002

- The Global Fund is established to boost the response to AIDS, TB and malaria in developing countries.
- Botswana begins Africa's first national AIDS treatment programme.
- The South African government approves AZT as post-exposure prophylaxis (PEP) for women who have been raped.

2003

- Drug manufacturers lower the prices of antiretroviral drugs for resource-poor countries.
- WHO launches the "3 by 5" initiative to widen access to AIDS treatment in developing countries.
- Of 4.1 million people in sub-Saharan Africa who need treatment for HIV, just over 1% are accessing it.

2004

- President Bush launches PEPFAR, a $15 billion AIDS initiative with 12 focus African countries.
- The South African government begins funding antiretroviral treatment for AIDS patients.
- Uganda has reduced its HIV prevalence by 70% since the early 1990s.
- The G8 summit leaders promise to double aid to Africa and to ensure near universal access to antiretroviral treatment worldwide by 2010.
- Nelson Mandela announces that his eldest son has died of AIDS.

2006

- 28% of people in sub-Saharan Africa who need treatment for HIV are receiving it.
- Large studies of male circumcision reveal firm evidence that the procedure reduces the risk of HIV infection.

2007

- Botswana has succeeded in cutting its mother-to-child transmission rate to under 4% - a rate comparable with the USA and Western Europe.

2008

Botswana has succeeded in cutting its mother-to-child

2009

Botswana has succeeded in cutting its mother-to-child

2010

Botswana has succeeded in cutting its mother-to-child

2011

Botswana has succeeded in cutting its mother-to-child

2012

Botswana has succeeded in cutting its mother-to-child

2013

Botswana has succeeded in cutting its mother-to-child

2014

Botswana has succeeded in cutting its mother-to-child

CHAPTER NINE

HIV/AIDS PREVALENCES

International statistics on HIV/AIDS

The number of new HIV infections has declined globally by 21% since the estimated peak of the epidemic in 1997

- 2.3 million people were newly infected with HIV worldwide in 2012
- In some parts of the world (particularly within Sub-Saharan Africa) between 15-28% of the population are living with HIV

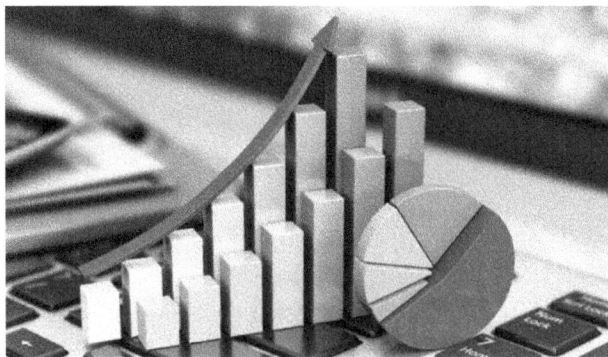

Source: NACA Website; April, 2017

People living with HIV globally

- 35.3 million people living with HIV worldwide
- 47% of people living with HIV worldwide are women

- 1.6 million AIDS-related deaths

New HIV cases around the globe in 2012

- 2.3 million people diagnosed with HIV
- 6,300 new HIV infections a day
- 260 000 new HIV infections among children
- 95% are in low- and middle-income countriesmon

Worldwide HIV & AIDS Statistics

Global HIV/AIDS estimates, end of 2013

The latest statistics on the world epidemic of AIDS & HIV were published by UNAIDS/WHO in July 2008, and refer to the end of 2013.

	Estimate	Range
People living with HIV/AIDS in 2013	33.0 million	30.3-36.1 million
Adults living with HIV/AIDS in 2013	30.8 million	28.2-34.0 million
Women living with HIV/AIDS in 2013	15.5 million	14.2-16.9 million
Children living with HIV/AIDS in 2013	2.0 million	1.9-2.3 million
People newly infected with HIV in 2013	2.7 million	2.2-3.2 million
Children newly infected with HIV in 2013	0.37 million	0.33-0.41 million

AIDS deaths in 2013   2.0 million   1.8-2.3 million

Child AIDS deaths in 2013   0.27 million 0.25-0.29 million

More than 30 million people have died of AIDS since 1981.

Africa has 13.6 million AIDS orphans.

At the end of 2007, women accounted for 50% of all adults living with HIV worldwide, and for 59% in sub-Saharan Africa.

Young people (under 25 years old) account for half of all new HIV infections worldwide.

In developing and transitional countries, 9.7 million people are in immediate need of life-saving AIDS drugs; of these, only 2.99 million (31%) are receiving the drugs.

Global summary of the AIDS epidemic   2015

Number of people living with HIV in 2015		
Total	36.7 million	[34.0 million – 39.8 million]
Adults	34.9 million	[32.4 million – 37.9 million]
Women (15+)	17.8 million	[16.4 million – 19.4 million]
Children (<15 years)	1.8 million	[1.5 million – 2.0 million]

People newly infected with HIV in 2015		
Total	2.1 million	[1.8 million – 2.4 million]
Adults	1.9 million	[1.7 million – 2.2 million]
Children (<15 years)	150 000	[110 000 – 190 000]

AIDS deaths in 2015		
Total	1.1 million	[940 000 – 1.3 million]
Adults	1.0 million	[840 000 – 1.2 million]
Children (<15 years)	110 000	[84 000 – 130 000]

WHO – HIV department | June 15, 2016   World Health Organization UNAIDS unicef

Global trends

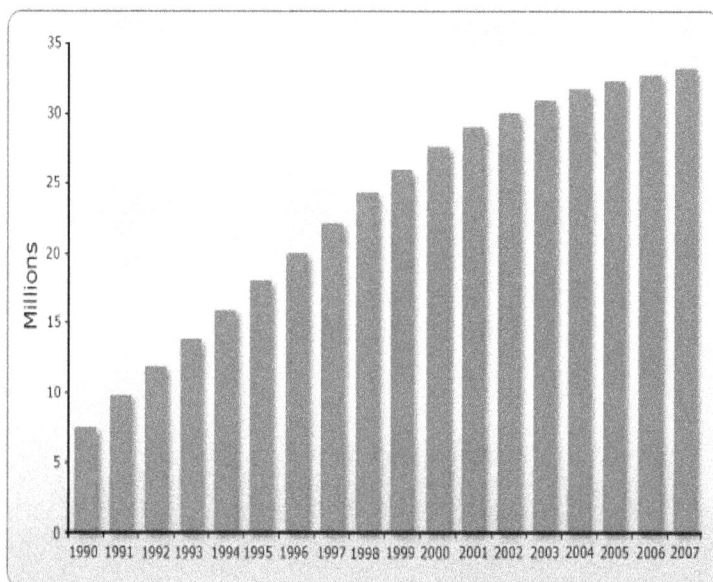

The number of people living with HIV has risen from around 8 million in 1990 to 33 million today, and is still growing. Around 67% of people living with HIV are in sub-Saharan Africa.

Regional statistics for HIV & AIDS.

Region	Adults & children living with HIV/AIDS	Adults & children newly infected	Adult prevalence*	Deaths of adults & children
Sub-Saharan Africa	22.0 million	1.9 million	5.0%	1.5 million
North Africa & Middle East	380,000	40,000	0.3%	27,000

Region				
Asia	5 million	380,000	0.3%	380,000
Oceania	74,000	13,000	0.4%	1,000
Latin America	1.7 million	140,000	0.5%	63,000
Caribbean	230,000	20,000	1.1%	14,000
Eastern Europe & Central Asia	1.5 million	110,000	0.8%	58,000
North America, Western & Central Europe	2.0 million	81,000	0.4%	31,000
Global Total	33.0 million	2.7 million	0.8%	2.0 million

Proportion of adults aged 15-49 who were living with HIV/AIDS

During 2007 more than two and a half million adults and children became infected with HIV (Human Immunodeficiency Virus), the virus that causes AIDS. By the end of the year, an estimated 33 million people worldwide were living with HIV/AIDS. The year also saw two million deaths from AIDS, despite recent improvements in access to antiretroviral treatment.

Notes

Adults are defined as men and women aged 15 or above, unless specified otherwise.

Children orphaned by AIDS are defined as people aged under 18 who are alive and have lost one or both parents to AIDS.

All the statistics on this page should be interpreted with caution because they are estimates.

Worldwide HIV & AIDS Statistics Commentary

Number of people living with HIV

According to estimates from the UNAIDS 2008 Report on the global AIDS epidemic, around 30.8 million adults and 2 million children were living with HIV at the end of 2007.

Number of people infected during 2007, and the number of deaths

During 2007, some 2.7 million people became infected with the human immunodeficiency virus (HIV), which causes AIDS.

The year also saw 2 million deaths from AIDS - a high global total, despite antiretroviral (ARV) therapy, which reduced AIDS-related deaths among those who received it. The number of deaths probably peaked around 2005, and has since declined only slightly.

How people become infected with HIV

Globally, around 11% of HIV infections are among babies who acquire the virus from their mothers; 10% result from injecting drug use; 5-10% is due to sex between men; and 5-10% occurs in healthcare settings. Sex between men and women accounts for the remaining proportion – around two thirds of new infections.

Young people affected by HIV and AIDS

Around half of the people who acquire HIV become infected before they turn 25 and typically die of the life-threatening illnesses called AIDS before their 35th birthday. By the end of 2007, the epidemic had left behind 15 million AIDS orphans, defined as those aged under 18 who have lost one or both parents to AIDS. These orphans are vulnerable to poverty, exploitation and themselves becoming infected with HIV. They are often forced to leave the education system and find work, and sometimes to care for younger siblings or head a family.

In 2007, around 370,000 children aged 14 or younger became infected with HIV. Over 90% of newly infected children are babies born to women with HIV, who acquire the virus during pregnancy, labour or delivery, or through their mother's breast milk. Almost nine-tenths of such transmissions occur in sub-Saharan Africa. Africa's lead in mother-to-child transmission of HIV is firmer than ever despite the evidence that HIV ultimately impairs women's fertility; once infected, a woman can be expected to bear 20% fewer children than she otherwise would. Drugs are available to minimize the dangers of mother-to-child HIV transmission, but these are still often not reaching the places where they are most needed.

HIV/AIDS around the world

The overwhelming majority of people with HIV, some 95% of the global total, live in the developing world. The proportion is set to grow even further as infection rates continue to rise in countries where poverty, poor health care systems and limited resources for prevention and care fuel the spread of the virus.

The chart on the right shows the distribution of people living with HIV around the world, according to 2007 data.

High-income countries

The total number of people living with HIV continues to rise in high-income countries, largely due to widespread access to ARV therapy, which prolongs the lives of HIV+ people. This increases the pool of HIV-infected people who are able to transmit the virus onwards. It is estimated that 1.2 million people are living with HIV in North America and 730,000 in Western and Central Europe.

In these two regions, AIDS claimed approximately 31,000 lives in 2007. The rate of AIDS-related deaths has been cut substantially through use of ARV medicines. There is mounting evidence that prevention activities in several high-income countries are not keeping pace with the spread of HIV and that in some places they are falling behind. Such shortcomings are most evident where HIV is found mainly among marginalized groups of the population, such as drug users, immigrants and refugees.

AVERT.org has pages about HIV and AIDS in the USA and in the UK, plus statistics pages covering many high income countries, including Australia, Canada and Western Europe.

United States of America

In the United States, the burden of HIV and AIDS is not evenly distributed across states and regions. In most areas of the country, HIV is concentrated in urban areas, so states reporting more diagnoses or higher rates of persons living with diagnosed HIV infection or ever classified as AIDS usually contain major metropolitan areas. But in the South, larger percentages of diagnoses are in smaller metropolitan and nonmetropolitan areas. Understanding the places and populations that are most affected by HIV and AIDS allows the federal government to allocate its resources to the geographic areas where they are needed most, while still supporting a basic level of HIV education and prevention for everyone across the country.

HIV Diagnoses, by Race/Ethnicity, Region, and State

Most HIV diagnoses in 2015 were among blacks/African Americans,[a] Hispanics/Latinos,[b] or whites, reflecting the majority population groups of the United States.

The rates (per 100,000 people) of HIV diagnoses in 2015 were 16.8 in the South, 11.6 in the Northeast, 9.8 in the West, and 7.6 in the Midwest.[c]

Rates of HIV Diagnoses Among Adults and Adolescents in the US in 2015, by State

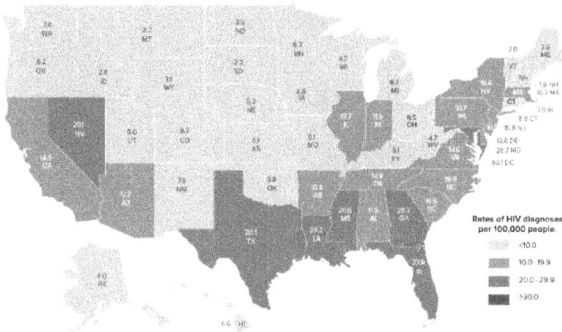

Source: CDC. Diagnoses of HIV infection in the United States and dependent areas, 2015. **HIV Surveillance Report** *2016; 27.*

Diagnoses of HIV Infection in the US in 2015, by Race/Ethnicity and Region of Residence

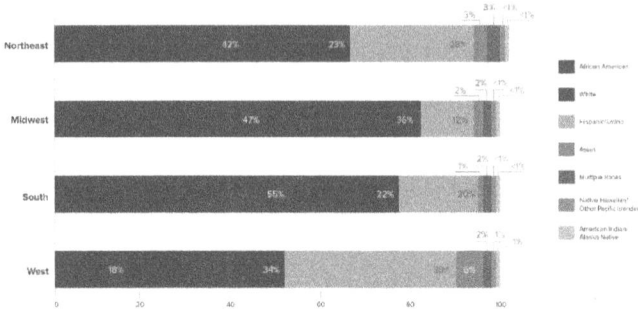

Source: CDC. Diagnoses of HIV infection in the United States and dependent areas, 2015. **HIV Surveillance Report 2016; 27.**

Lifetime Risk of HIV, by State

Overall, an American has a 1 in 99 chance of being diagnosed with HIV at some point in his or her life. But that lifetime risk is greater for people living in the South than in other regions of the country. The lifetime risk of HIV diagnosis is highest in the District of Columbia, followed by Maryland, Georgia, Florida, Louisiana, New York, Texas, New Jersey, Mississippi, South Carolina, North Carolina, Delaware, and Alabama.

Lifetime Risk of HIV Diagnosis, by State

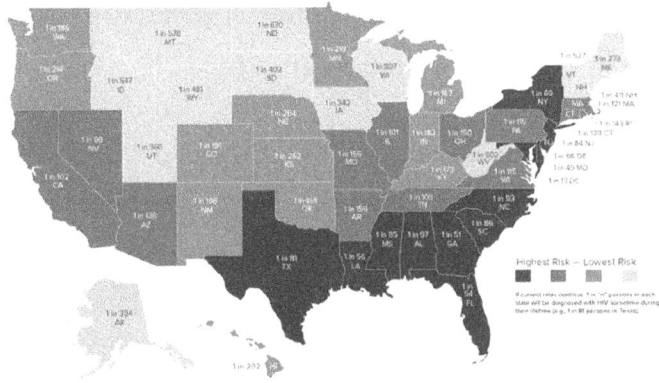

Source: CDC. Lifetime risk of HIV diagnosis [press release]. February 23, 2016.

Sub-Saharan Africa

The area in Africa south of the Sahara desert, known as sub-Saharan Africa, is by far the worst-affected in the world by the AIDS epidemic. The region has just over 10% of the world's population, but is home to 67% of all people living with HIV. An estimated 1.9 million adults and children became infected with HIV during 2007. This brought the total number of people living with HIV/AIDS in the region to 22 million by the end of the year. HIV prevalence varies considerably across this region - ranging from less than 1% in Madagascar to over 25% in Swaziland.

HIV prevalence (the proportion of people living with HIV) appears to have fallen slightly in this region over recent years because the number of new infections is exceeded by the number of deaths each year. However, the total number of people living with HIV is still rising because of overall population growth.

In sub-Saharan Africa, AIDS killed approximately 1.5 million people in 2007. Average survival in the absence of treatment is around 10 years after infection. ARV drugs can dramatically extend survival, allowing many years of healthy life, but these remain unavailable to most Africans.

Unlike women in most other regions in the world, African women are considerably more likely - at least 1.4 times - to be infected with HIV than men. There are a number of reasons why female prevalence is higher than male in this region, including the greater efficiency of male-to-female HIV transmission through sex and the younger age at initial infection for women.

Eastern Europe and Central Asia

The AIDS epidemic in Eastern Europe and Central Asia is rapidly expanding. Some 110,000 people were infected with HIV in 2007, bringing the total number of people living with the virus to around 1.5 million. Only a small proportion of HIV+ people in these areas can hope to receive ARV medication, so the AIDS death rate - which was around 58,000 in 2007 - is higher than it might otherwise be.

Worst affected are the Russian Federation, Ukraine, and the Baltic states (Estonia, Latvia, and Lithuania), but HIV continues to spread in Belarus, Moldova and Kazakhstan, while more recent epidemics are now evident in Kyrgyzstan and Uzbekistan. It is now estimated that around 940,000 people are living with HIV in the Russian Federation.

Asia

Until recently it was thought that India was home to around 5.7 million people living with HIV - more than any other country in the world. In July 2007 this estimate was revised to between 2 million and 3.1 million, based on better data including the results of a national household survey.

Because of the major revision of the Indian estimate, the number of people living with HIV in the whole of Asia is now thought to be substantially less than the figure published by UNAIDS in late 2006. The current estimate is around 5 million.

National adult prevalence is still under 1% in the majority of this region's countries. However some Asian countries are very large and national averages may obscure serious epidemics in some smaller provinces and states. Although national adult HIV prevalence in India, for example, is below 1%, some states have an estimated prevalence well above this level. Other countries with large numbers of people living with HIV include China (700,000), Thailand (610,000) and Viet Nam (290,000).

North Africa and the Middle East

The notion that this region has sidestepped the global epidemic - perhaps due to strict rules governing sexual behaviour - is not supported by the latest estimates, which indicate that 40,000 people acquired an HIV infection in 2007, bringing the total number of people living with HIV/AIDS in the Middle East and North Africa to an estimated 380,000. AIDS killed a further 27,000 people in 2007.

Latin America and the Caribbean

An estimated 1.7 million people are living with HIV in Latin America and the Caribbean, including the estimated 140,000 who became infected during 2007. Around 63,000 people died of AIDS in the same year.

All the main modes of transmission exist in most countries, along with significant levels of risky behaviour - such as early sexual debut, unprotected sex with multiple partners and the use of unclean drug-injecting equipment. The largest HIV epidemic is in Brazil, where around 730,000 people are living with the virus, though the death rate has fallen due to widespread access to treatment. Adult HIV prevalence in five countries is more than 2% - higher than anywhere else outside sub-Saharan Africa.

The future

Future projections of the extent of the HIV/AIDS epidemic cannot be made with any precision; what happens next will depend on what action is taken. In some scenarios, governments and societies mount a very vigorous and wide-ranging response which recognizes AIDS as much more than just a health issue, and so HIV prevalence eventually decreases; in other projections, good intentions fail to deliver anything more than short-term and fractured responses in the worst-affected countries, and the number of people living with HIV soars.

The World Health Organization does not publish predictions of HIV prevalence, but it does project AIDS mortality. Provided antiretroviral therapy access continues to grow at the current rate, the annual number of deaths due to AIDS is expected to peak at around 2.4 million in 2012, and then to decline to 1.2 million in 2030. Yet even in this scenario, AIDS will remain one of the ten leading causes of death globally.

Minimizing the impact of HIV will require massive responses at the national and international level:

- People need to challenge the myths and misconceptions about human sexuality that translate into dangerous sexual practices.
- Work and legislation is needed to reduce prejudice felt by HIV+ people around the world and the

discrimination that prevents people from "coming out" as being HIV positive.

- HIV prevention initiatives need to be increased, people across the world need to be made aware of the dangers, the risks, and the ways they can protect themselves.
- Condom promotion and supply needs to be increased, and the appropriate sexual health education needs to be provided to young people before they reach an age where they become sexually active.
- Medication and support needs to be provided to people who are already HIV+, so that they can live longer and more productive lives, support their families, and avoid transmitting the virus onwards.
- Support and care needs to be provided for those children who have already been orphaned by AIDS, so that they can grow up safely, without experiencing poverty, exploitation, and themselves falling prey to HIV.

Sub Saharan Africa HIV & AIDS Statistics

An estimated 22 million adults and children were living with HIV in sub-Saharan Africa at the end of 2007.

During that year, an estimated 1.5 million Africans died from AIDS. The epidemic has left behind some 11.6 million orphaned African children.

The estimated number of adults and children living with HIV/AIDS, the number of deaths from AIDS, and the number of living orphans in individual countries in sub-Saharan Africa at the end of 2007 are shown below.

Country	People living with HIV/AIDS	Adult (15-49) rate %	Women with HIV/AIDS	Children with HIV/AIDS	AIDS deaths	Orphans due to AIDS
Angola	190,000	2.1	110,000	17,000	11,000	50,000
Benin	64,000	1.2	37,000	5,400	3,300	29,000
Botswana	300,000	23.9	170,000	15,000	11,000	95,000
Burkina Faso	130,000	1.6	61,000	10,000	9,200	100,000
Burundi	110,000	2.0	53,000	15,000	11,000	120,000
Cameroon	540,000	5.1	300,000	45,000	39,000	300,000
Central African Republic	160,000	6.3	91,000	14,000	11,000	72,000
Chad	200,000	3.5	110,000	19,000	14,000	85,000
Comoros	<200	<0.1	<100	<100	<100	<100
Congo	120,000	3.5	43,000	6,600	6,400	69,000
Côte d'Ivoire	480,000	3.9	250,000	52,000	38,000	420,000
Dem. Republic of Congo	400,000-500,000	1.2-1.5	210,000-270,000	37,000-52,000	24,000-34,000	270,000-380,000

Djibouti	16,000	3.1	8,700	1,100	1,100	5,200
Equatorial Guinea	11,000	3.4	5,900	<1,000	<1,000	4,800
Eritrea	38,000	1.3	21,000	3,100	2,600	18,000
Ethiopia	980,000	2.1	530,000	92,000	67,000	650,000
Gabon	49,000	5.9	27,000	2,300	2,300	18,000
Gambia	8,200	0.9	4,500	<1,000	<1,000	2,700
Ghana	260,000	1.9	150,000	17,000	21,000	160,000
Guinea	87,000	1.6	48,000	6,300	4,500	25,000
Guinea-Bissau	16,000	1.8	8,700	1,500	1,100	6,200
Kenya	1,500,000-2,000,000	7.1-8.5	800,000-1,100,000	130,000-180,000	85,000-130,000	990,000-1,400,000
Lesotho	270,000	23.2	150,000	12,000	18,000	110,000
Liberia	35,000	1.7	19,000	3,100	2,300	15,000
Madagascar	14,000	0.1	3,400	<500	<1,000	3,400
Malawi	930,000	11.9	490,000	91,000	68,000	560,000
Mali	100,000	1.5	56,000	9,400	5,800	44,000
Mauritania	14,000	0.8	3,900	<500	<1,000	3,000
Mauritius	13,000	1.7	3,800	<100	<1,000	<500
Mozambique	1,500,000	12.5	810,000	100,000	81,000	400,000

Namibia	200,000	15.3	110,000	14,000	5,100	66,000
Niger	60,000	0.8	17,000	3,200	4,000	25,000
Nigeria	2,600,000	3.1	1,400,000	220,000	170,000	1,200,000
Rwanda	150,000	2.8	78,000	19,000	7,800	220,000
Senegal	67,000	1.0	38,000	3,100	1,800	8,400
Sierra Leone	55,000	1.7	30,000	4,000	3,300	16,000
Somalia	24,000	0.5	6,700	<1,000	1,600	8,800
South Africa	5,700,000	18.1	3,200,000	280,000	350,000	1,400,000
Swaziland	190,000	26.1	100,000	15,000	10,000	56,000
Togo	130,000	3.3	69,000	10,000	9,100	68,000
Uganda	1,000,000	6.7	520,000	110,000	91,000	1,000,000
United Rep. Of Tanzania	940,000	5.4	480,000	130,000	77,000	1,200,000
Zambia	1,100,000	15.2	560,000	95,000	56,000	600,000
Zimbabwe	1,300,000	15.3	680,000	120,000	140,000	1,000,000
Total sub-Saharan Africa	22,000,000	5.0	12,000,000	1,800,000	1,500,000	11,600,000

Notes

Adults in this page are defined as men and women aged over 15, unless specified otherwise.

Children are defined as people under the age of 15, whilst orphans are people aged under 18 who have lost one or both parents to AIDS.

CONCLUSION

Indeed, we've discussed extensively on HIV/ AIDS. It will be wise to emphasize that HIV/AIDS is a pandemic, which we must all work towards its amelioration. Remember, we should show love to PLHA and PABA. Lack of adequate and necessary information could have led to their being infected and or affected.

To be HIV positive is not a crime, we should not allow it to progress to AIDS which is the terminal stage of HIV: if not managed. To be infected with HIV does not mean that you are doomed; it's all about your state of mind and how you take care of yourself. "If your feel sick, you are sick". Your state of mind masterminds and determines what happens to your bio-physiological functionality. Don't be deceived most PLHA died because of the way they were treated by our society. They are not outcasts; do not treat them like that. With the little resources, they can take care of themselves.

At this juncture, I think it's pertinent to advice you to go for HIV test. If you are afraid of people knowing your status, Self Test Kits are there for you, it is wise to know your status and be counseled on how to live your life, than not knowing your status and die of AIDS.

Remember, it is not enough to know about HIV/AIDS. It is important to have accurate and complete information and also to use them wisely to protect one from this life wasting scourge.

Do not be deceived, AIDS is real and currently has no cure. It terminal point is death if not properly managed. Meanwhile, HIV is different from AIDS. To be HIV positive does not mean that you must have AIDS. So let's help our society by passing HIV/AIDS information correctly. **Pass it on please.**

REFERENCES

VOA   African News, Tuesday,   July 6, 2007.

John Christian, (Unpublished). Bundi Group.

Associate Professor McCain. University of Jos.

TIME, February 22, 2006.

International Project for Affordable Therapy for HIV: P. O. Box 691068 Los Angels, CA 90069. USA.

aidsrestherapy.biomedcentral.com/articles/10.1186/s12981 -016-0118-7

who.int/hiv/data/en/

ACRONYMS

- **HIV** -Human Immunodeficiency Virus.
- **AIDS** -Acquired Immune Deficiency Syndrome.
- **PLHA** -People Living With HIV/AIDS.
- **PABA** -People Affected By AIDS.
- **OI** -Opportunistic Infections.
- **RH** -Reproduction Health.
- **ARH** -Adolescences Reproductive Health.
- **ARV** -Anti-Retroviral Drugs.
- **TB** -Tuberculosis.
- **BCR** -Bundi Counseling/Referral Center.
- **RNA** -Ribonucleic Acid.
- **DNA** -Deoxonuclecis Acid.
- **HCT** -HIV Counseling and Testing.
- **OVC** -Orphans and Vulnerable Children.
- **BCC** -Behaviour Change Communication.
- **STI** -Sexually Transmitted Infection
- **TB** -Tuberculosis
- **PTB** -Pulmonary TB
- **ART** -Antiretroviral therapy
- **ATT** -Anti-tuberculosis therapy
- **LTBI** -Latent TB infection
- **TST** -Tuberculin sensitivity test
- **IGRA** -Interferon gamma releases assay
- **CXR** -Chest X-ray
- **AFB** -Acid fast bacillus
- **M.Tb** -Mycobacterium tuberculosis
- **MGIT** -Mycobacterial growth indicator tube
- **NAAT** -Nucleic acid amplification test

- **VEGF** -Vascular endothelial growth factor
- **ADA** -Adenosine deaminase
- **LAM** -Lipoarabinomannan
- **LPA**-Line probe assay
- **INH**-Isoniazid
- **IPT** -INH preventive therapy
- **STCI** -Standards of TB care in India
- **DOT** -Directly observed therapy
- **ARR** -Acquired rifampicin resistance
- **NIRT** -National Institute for Research in tuberculosis
- **CD** -Cluster of differentiation
- **MDR** -Multidrug resistant
- **XDR** -Extensively drug resistance
- **IRIS** -Immune reconstitution inflammatory syndrome
- **MMP** -Matrix metallo-proteinases
- **INSHI** -International network for the study of HIV associated IRIS

DO YOU KNOW THAT...

You might be thinking that you are healthy and cannot have this scourge but that is not true. HIV is not a respecter of any person neither does it know any boundary. It has nothing to do with class rather behaviour.

To safeguard your future and that of the unborn babies, you have to go for HCT. If your test result is negative, you will than take caution so as not to be infected with the virus. But if the test result is positive, you will be counseled on how to live your life so as to prevent you from having AIDS.

To ensure the concept of confidentiality which will ameliorate most psychological trauma that is associated with the endemic, the need to use self test kit emanated.

Go for HCT today. "Your life is a priceless Jewel which can hardly be replaced. You ought to handle it with care".

Remember, counseling principles are:

- Individualization
- Effective communication of feelings
- Controlling emotional involvement
- Acceptance of client's situation
- Non-judgment attitudes
- Client self determination

- Confidentiality
- Trustworthy
- Politeness
- Empathy

ABOUT THE AUTHOR

Kalu, **Prince-Iroha,**A Professional Social Worker, Research and HIV Management Consultantholds Graduate and Post-graduate Degrees from the University of Calabar, Nigeria; Heis a member of The International Network of Social Workers; International AIDS Society; The Network for Social Work Management; International HIV/AIDS Alliance; and Social Problem Amelioration Institute. He is also a licensee and an International Master Trainer of the Applied Scholastics International, 11755 Riverview Drive, St. Louis, Missouri USA. He has the status of UNICEF HIV/AIDS trained Educator and, a Consultant on Social Problem Amelioration and HIV/AIDS Educators.

He started his career with BUNDI International Diagnostic, Nigeria where he was Head of HIV Counseling/Referral Unit, before setting up his own firm (Praik-Applied Nigeria). He was a Mentor of the Federal Government of Nigeria YouWin Program.

Kalu, Prince-Iroha enjoys travelling, reading, writing,voluntary services and giving lives new meaning. A member of the Believers Loveworld International, he hails from Abia Ohafia in Abia State, Nigeria. He has toured several countries in the discharge of his duties (especially in the field of Study Technology). Presently, he is the Program Director of Praik-Applied Nigeria; and as well, the Project Director of Abia State Grassroots' Sports

Development Initiatives (ABGRASOD), which is a Collaborative Project of Abia State Government and Praik-Applied Nigeria.

He is happily married to his heart desire, Mrs. Hope Prince-Iroha and is blessed with beautiful children.

ABOUT THE BOOK

As the then head of the HIV/AIDS Counseling/ Referral Department of BUNDI International Diagnostics, I was in constant touch with those who stand the risk of HIV infection, those who are infected with the virus and those who are living with HIV/AIDS. I had first-hand knowledge of the test results of client. This, more than any other factor prompted me to write the book "HIV does not mean Death. The Socio-Psychological perspective of HIV/AIDS: why most people Die of AIDS".

The bible says that out of the abundance of the heart the mouth speaks (*Matt. 12:34b*), I have seen much and been highly challenged so I speak. This explains the many words and phrases that I used for the title of this book. Perhaps a less burdened person would have used fewer words. Also, the chapter headings' equally portray this heaviness of heart.

The purpose of this book is to expose the reader to the global realities of HIV/AIDS. To achieve these, we have five main objectives, namely:

1. To create awareness and educate the reader about HIV/AIDS

2. To convince the reader to know his or her status

and, in so doing, to live positively.

3.   To reveal to the reader the impact of HIV/AIDS to the individual, the community and the whole nation.

4.   To call the reader to action to take proactive measures against HIV/AIDS and to shun stigma and discrimination against people living with HIV/AIDS.

5.   To give an adequate guide towards an effective HIV Management and Mitigation.

The first four chapters of this book are devoted to awareness creation and education about HIV/AIDS. From the first chapter I brought in my training in psychology and as a counselor to bear by bringing the reader to the knowledge of the power of the mind over the body of the sufferer of any ailment. Still in the first chapter I used poetry to expose to the reader the stark reality of the phenomenon of HIV/AIDS and the absurdity of (casual, unprotected and unsafe) sexual pleasure which leads to life-long pain. At the end of this poem, I call for actions to end the pandemic. The action is to get tested, and the second action is to stop stigma and discrimination against people living with AIDS.

Next, I cut out a large space to educate people about HIV/AIDS and give an overview of HIV infection and AIDS. My account of HIV transmission is lucid, emphasizing the main source of infection as sexual intercourse with an infected person, sharing sharp skin instrument with an infected person, receiving blood from an infected person and vertical transmission from an infected mother to her child during pregnancy, at birth, or breast feedings.

There is a detailed account of signs and symptoms; and diagnoses of HIV/AIDS. There is also a section on treatment of HIV/AIDS. Here,I demonstrated my ability to do extensive research. I am a social scientist, however, for the purpose of this book and for my readers I delved into the field of pharmacology and toxicology to provide a list of antiretroviral drugs, their classes, uses, mechanisms of action and side effects. There is a brief section on opportunistic infection that afflict people living with HIV/AIDS.

Next is the behavioral link of HIV infection. There is also a little exposition on the mode of replication of HIV and how this eventually leads to AIDS.Window period which complicate the diagnosis of HIV infectionalso has a section.

In the next Chapter, we discussed the socio-psychological impact of HIV/AIDS. Pre-and post-tests are the antidotes to early deaths that were then rampant among people living with HIV.

The closing Chapter talks about the impacts of HIV/AIDS demographically and the call to action.

www.ingramcontent.com/pod-product-compliance
Lightning Source LLC
Chambersburg PA
CBHW032352280326
41935CB00008B/541